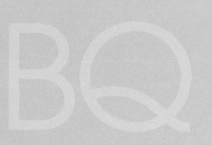

Praise for *The Beauty Quotient Formula*

"Dr. Tornambe offers helpful alternatives to those people who would prefer not to go under the knife but are still hoping to look better and feel better at any age."

— **Joan Rivers**, comedian

"This book is a must read for anyone who might seek personal, and perhaps, physical and psychological changes in their lives."

— **Raymond LaRaja, M.D.**, clinical professor of surgery at Mt. Sinai Medical School and former clinical professor of surgery at New York University Medical School

THE BEAUTY QUOTIENT

FORMULA

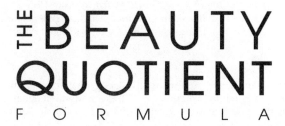

THE BEAUTY QUOTIENT FORMULA

HOW TO FIND YOUR OWN
BEAUTY QUOTIENT
TO LOOK YOUR BEST—
NO MATTER WHAT YOUR AGE

ROBERT M. TORNAMBE, M.D., F.A.C.S.
with Karen Moline

HAY HOUSE, INC.
Carlsbad, California • New York City
London • Sydney • Johannesburg
Vancouver • Hong Kong • New Delhi

Published and distributed in the United States by: Hay House, Inc.: www.hayhouse.com • *Published and distributed in Australia by:* Hay House Australia Pty. Ltd.: www.hayhouse.com.au • *Published and distributed in the United Kingdom by:* Hay House UK, Ltd.: www.hayhouse.co.uk • *Published and distributed in the Republic of South Africa by:* Hay House SA (Pty), Ltd.: www.hayhouse.co.za • *Distributed in Canada by:* Raincoast: www.raincoast.com • *Published in India by:* Hay House Publishers India: www.hayhouse.co.in

Design: Jami Goddess

Interior photos: Clara Bow – Hulton Archive/Getty Images; Katharine Hepburn – Clarence Sinclair Bull/Hulton Archive/Getty Images; Ingrid Bergman – John Kobal Foundation/Hulton Archive/Getty Images; Audrey Hepburn – Allan Grant/Time & Life Pictures/Getty Images; Twiggy – Michael Ochs Archives/Getty Images; Bette Midler – CBS Photo Archive/Hulton Archive/Getty Images; Tina Turner – GAB Archive/Redferns/Getty Images; Kate Moss – Dave Allocca/Time & Life Pictures/ Getty Images; Michelle Yeoh – Evan Agostini/Getty Images Entertainment/Getty Images; Appendix D – Virgil Wong

    The author of this book does not dispense medical advice or prescribe the use of any technique as a form of treatment for physical, emotional, or medical problems without the advice of a physician, either directly or indirectly. The intent of the author is only to offer information of a general nature to help you in your quest for emotional and spiritual well-being. In the event you use any of the information in this book for yourself, which is your constitutional right, the author and the publisher assume no responsibility for your actions.

Library of Congress Cataloging-in-Publication Data

Tornambe, Robert M. (Robert Milo)
 The beauty quotient formula : how to find your own beauty quotient to look your best- no matter what your age / Robert M. Tornambe. -- 1st ed.
    p. cm.
 Includes index.

 ISBN 978-1-4019-2451-5 (hardcover : alk. paper) 1. Beauty, Personal. 2. Body image. I. Title.
 HQ1219.T67 2010
 646.7'2--dc22

                                      2009045604ISBN: 978-1-4019-2451-5

13 12 11 10   4 3 2 1
1st edition, April 2010

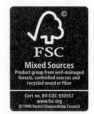

FSC
Mixed Sources
Product group from well-managed forests, controlled sources and recycled wood or fiber
Cert no. BV-COC-930557
www.fsc.org
© 1996 Forest Stewardship Council

To My Father

His wisdom, kindness, and generosity provided
a beacon of integrity to guide his four sons
through life, long after his passing.

CONTENTS

Introduction

Beautiful? For whom? Why, for myself, of course.

— Colette

One night when I was out to dinner with some friends, I glanced over to a nearby table and saw an elderly woman in a wheelchair, choking. She had stopped breathing and was turning blue, so I jumped from my seat and ran over to help. I identified myself as a doctor, and my friends and I got her out of the wheelchair and performed the Heimlich maneuver. She quickly recovered, and her daughter, with whom she'd been eating, thanked me profusely.

"What kind of doctor are you?" she asked.

"I'm a plastic surgeon," I replied.

"Oh, really?" she asked, looking at me aghast. *"With that nose?"*

That was her thank-you for me saving her mother's life—not the nicest, I'll admit, but it got me thinking. I like my nose the way it is, and I like the wrinkles on my forehead. Quite frankly, I'm happy with the way I look now. But the people who come to me for plastic surgery aren't, even when they have physical features that would be considered more beautiful than my less-than-svelte nose or my wrinkled forehead. What, precisely, are my patients seeking?

I've spent more than 25 years examining and operating on thousands of patients, listening to their dreams, hopes, and desires. As a physician and surgeon, I wanted to offer my patients as many options as possible, so they could choose which was healthiest for them. This quest led me to develop a comprehensive approach to beauty that looks at more than the physical—one that provides solutions to beauty concerns without having to go under the knife. I call this system BQ, or Beauty Quotient. It looks at that indefinable something that makes one person's face, which might not be considered classically beautiful, work so well, while others with perfect features seem somehow lacking. Although beauty is truly an *indefinable* characteristic—one that's always going to remain in the eye of the beholder—my spin on this was not to look for the flaws, but to look for and accentuate all the inimitable factors that make each person unique.

A person's BQ rating—the higher the better—comes from a combination of factors. Having a slightly-too-large nose, an overbite, and sparkling eyes coupled with a certain radiance and vitality, for example, can mesh together in a unique harmony. It is this interplay that makes someone beautiful or homely—not their physical features alone.

After all, how many times have you met someone strikingly beautiful or handsome, but after five minutes of conversation, you suddenly realize that this person no longer has such a zing? Something about their personality became off-putting to you—perhaps an offhand comment, a gesture, how they behave, or the scent of their perfume. Any of these factors can instantly increase or decrease a person's BQ according to *your* perception of them.

Take, for example, my perception of news anchor Connie Chung. I met her years ago when I was called to a New York City emergency room to treat her husband, Maury Povich, who had sustained a facial laceration while working out. We spoke briefly on several occasions, and I remember thinking how exquisite she was—so much prettier in person than on TV. I soon realized that her unforced charm, wit, and lively personality, as well as her beauty (untouched by a scalpel) gave her a very high BQ score.

Another woman with an amazingly high BQ was Jacqueline Kennedy Onassis. One of my favorite memories is of a cloudy, crisp fall day, when I was out running around the Central Park reservoir and noticed a tall, slender woman running toward me. I couldn't quite make her out at first, and then as we were getting closer and closer, I noticed the cheekbones. Then the famous eyes. And then—oh my God, it really was her!

Even if this woman hadn't been Jackie O, I still would have remembered the aura she exuded. Normally, you don't think it's possible for someone to be charismatic when they're sweaty and wearing simple workout clothes, but there was just something magical about Jackie.

Unfortunately, many of the women sitting in my office haven't discovered that there is more to their BQ than mere good looks. Often, this is because they're too busy wishing they had someone else's nose or lips or flat belly. When assessing my patients, I work hard to focus on and accentuate the positives rather than looking for the flaws. What are those positives? What are my patients seeking?

The Beauty Quotient Formula is a study of what makes someone beautiful and a guide to living in a way that will increase your beauty. You learn about the interplay of the external and internal—realizing that although beauty isn't only skin deep, skin still matters. You will see that to reach your highest BQ, you must focus on all parts of your life: your psychological health, your physical health, and your personal presentation. This book will help you realize how many of these factors are directly under your control, and it will give you specific techniques to maximize your unique attributes to boost your BQ sky-high.

We begin by deconstructing the faces and personalities of some of the most famous faces of the last hundred years, and then learn the Beauty Quotient commandments, the core principles that will guide you through the BQ program. From there, you'll take the BQ Formula quiz, which will give you a unique BQ score. It will help you see your beauty strengths and weaknesses, and it will direct you to different sections of the book that will teach you how to capitalize on your positive attributes and tackle your liabilities. Armed with that knowledge, you can maximize your Beauty Quotient, and as your BQ score grows larger, your life will become more streamlined. You won't have to think about what you're wearing because everything in your closet will make you look good. You won't have to fuss with your skincare or makeup because you'll have an easy daily routine. You'll know exactly how to look your best at all times, even if you only have ten minutes to get ready before you fly out the door!

Remember, the BQ is subjective, so there will never be a *perfect* score. But as soon as you start to reassess your strengths as well as your flaws, you'll be able to raise your BQ higher than you dreamed possible.

PART I

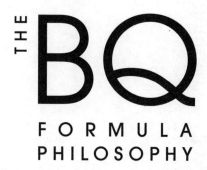

THE BQ
FORMULA
PHILOSOPHY

CHAPTER ONE

How to Deconstruct a Face to Discover Its BQ

How old is the quest for beauty? Oh, probably as old as civilization itself!

The Egyptians were as obsessed with beauty rituals as the ladies of today who pore over *Allure* magazine while getting one of their regular pedicures. Mummies have been found not just with gold and jewels but also with tweezers, pots of lip dyes, and recipes to combat wrinkles and pimples—after all, what royal Egyptian lady would have gone to the underworld without her upper lids lined with black kohl, her brows arched with antimony, or her body poisoned with the thick layer of pale lead paste carefully applied to her face?

Fortunately for the Egyptians, not every beauty treatment was toxic. During her reign circa 1400 B.C., Nefertiti was fond of a mixture of rainwater, natural limewater, and a clay paste made from Nile mud that she rubbed on her body with the aid of a pumice stone every morning. It was her unique exfoliation treatment, often followed with rehydrating and relaxing masks made from ostrich eggs, clay, oil, and milk.

The ancient Greeks left out the ostrich eggs, but they did make a long-lasting blush from crushed blackberries and figs. Take a look at this handy list of courtesan beauty aids, courtesy of Aristophanes: "Clippers, mirrors, grease-paint, soda, false hair, bands, ribbons, red paint, white lead, myrrh, pumice stones, vials, seaweed paint, chains for the neck, eye paint, gold ornaments for the hair, hair nets, girdles, mantillas, combs, earrings, ear-pendants, necklaces adorned with precious stones, bracelets, arm buckles, hair buckles, foot buckles, finger rings, beauty plasters, and hair supports."

The Greeks devised a formula to define beauty as a face that was two-thirds as long as it was wide; the brow one-third of the way down from the hairline and the mouth one-third way up from the chin.

The Roman writer Petronius took these measurements a bit further. According to his musings, the Roman ideal of beauty was a fair complexion, low forehead, and long eyebrows that met over the bridge of the nose. (Based on this description, Mexican artist Frida Kahlo would have likely found favor with Petronius.) A woman would need to have as much help as possible to combat the aftereffects of Roman cosmetology, which included such frightening beautifying processes as a face pack of sheep fat mixed with bread crumbs soaked in milk or crocodile excrement—to be left on all night!

Only slightly less hideous were Medieval dermatologic treatments, when skin was polished and whitened with a revolting concoction of arsenic sulfide, quick lime, ointments of hedgehog ashes, bats' blood, bees' wings, mercury, and slug slime. Hair was bleached with henna and animal innards. In the 1600s, makeup was made from highly toxic white lead mixed with chalk or in a paste of vinegar and egg whites. Interesting ingredients indeed, but on the other hand, sometimes I look at the long string of chemicals listed on the packaging of a 21st-century wrinkle cream, and I have to wonder how much has really changed!

Potions and concoctions aside, 21st-century discussions of beauty revolve around what we call AU, or aesthetic units. The eyes and the forehead are one AU. Your nose and midface, including your mouth, comprise your second AU. The chin and neck are the third AU. Each AU should flow seamlessly from one to another. It helps to think of these AUs as another way to group areas of the face, much as, during the Renaissance, Botticelli's formula for the glorious faces he painted was to break a face down into sevenths.

Still, AUs are helpful more from an anatomic point of view, or for considering symmetry, than they are for assessing what makes a beautiful face. For example, when plastic surgeons must reconstruct one part of the face after disfiguring cancer surgery or an automobile accident, the AUs assist in the planning of the reconstructive operations.

That these three AUs are interrelated is often something that plastic surgery patients don't understand at first. Which is why someone who wants her eyes done may look much better if she has a mini brow lift at the same time; someone who wants her nose reduced may look much better with a chin implant as well.

Striving to have a fairly uniform AU is pretty much the ideal of what Western society seems to identify as "classic" beauty. In fact, researchers in Australia have created computer software using an equation based on 14 facial measurements, 13 related ratios, and images of supermodels, actors, and more than 200 other women, so that when a photograph of a woman's face is fed into the program, it instantly returns a beauty rating of between one and ten.

According to the computer, beauty consists of even features; an oval-shaped face; large eyes; shapely and distinct cheekbones; a straight, small nose; well-shaped and defined lips; a round, firm chin; a long neck; round, high breasts; a trim waist; wide yet shapely hips; firm buttocks; long legs; and a slim figure. (And this "classic" beauty is usually classic only for Caucasians, not other races.)

Many women with similar AU measurements will have completely different BQ scores—being thought of as a classic beauty, with anatomically symmetrical AUs, doesn't automatically translate into a high BQ score. Sometimes AUs that are slightly distorted, such as large, full lips on a relatively small face, can be quite striking and attractive.

And some women whose features fall far from the notion of classic, often have some of the highest BQ scores possible. This was noted in an unusual way when computer scientists in Israel, as reported in the August 2008 proceedings of *Siggraph*, a computer graphics conference, developed what they called a "beautification engine." After 234 measurements were taken from faces, measuring the distance between features as well as other factors, they created a program based on their mathematical calculations of what was considered beautiful.

The results were fascinating. Asymmetrical eyes were evened out; large noses were reduced; chins grew stronger; cheekbones became more defined. Yet as the delicious little quirks of anatomy were erased entirely, the faces often looked worse or unnatural. Unusual beauties became merely pretty, which reinforces the basic BQ premise that it is the unique nuances of a woman's face—the traits and features that are *not* classically beautiful—that give her not just individuality but also beauty.

Most astonishing was the transformation of French superstar Brigitte Bardot, whose distinctively full upper lip and famous overbite were reduced—and in the click of a mouse her unique lusciousness disappeared. She became ordinary. So much for "beautification"!

Clearly, there is no such thing as the perfect nose or mouth or eyes or cheekbones, whether in real life or on a computer screen. This notion also supports my belief that running to a plastic surgeon in order to become more beautiful would, in some cases, be a huge mistake. Had Bardot changed the shape of her lips or gotten her teeth straightened, her BQ would have plummeted.

As legendary photographer Cecil Beaton once wrote about the dancer Irene Castle: "Like many works of art, it was not symmetry that made Mrs. Castle so alluring; she, too, proved that real beauty can often be irregular, and she created a dominant and striking personality from assets which any other woman at the time might well have regarded as liabilities."

With that description, Beaton perfectly described a woman with an exceptional BQ.

Let's take a look at some of the beauties of the 20th and 21st centuries, "deconstructing" their features to figure out what made their BQ so high. What you'll soon come to see is not only which of their features "work," but also how their style and attitude suffused every aspect of their appearance. As Diane Keaton once said in an interview, "You have to work with your flaws. You enhance them or hide them!"

FABLED, FAMOUS BEAUTIES

1920s—Clara Bow

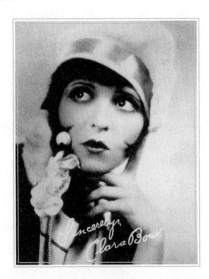

The original It Girl, Clara Bow became, for a short time at least, the epitome of flapper chic in the 1920s. But her face is fabled more for its artifice than for its proportions.

- Her eyes are large but her eyelids are heavy, leading to some serious drooping once the first blush of youth wears off.

- Her eyebrows had been shaved off and redrawn with a thick black pencil too dramatic for the small shape of her face.

- Her cheekbones are not defined.

- Her nose is wide, with a bulbous tip.

- Her chin is slightly receding.

- Her lips are her claim to fame—their "bee-stung" cupid's shape that was oh-so-desirable.

Long before lip fillers were invented, Clara Bow had one powerful pucker—and it was all hers. Accentuating her lips with dark lipstick would show clearly in the film stock of the silent films, and made them even more prominent and kissable.

Basically, Clara was a cute girl—not a gorgeous woman. But she knew how to transform herself from sweet to sultry by taking one feature and turning it into her claim to fame. It also didn't hurt that she had a come-hither sexuality, giving a hint of what the girl next door was really like when the lights went out.

Clara Bow's cute sexiness didn't age well though, and a few scant years after the heyday of flapper chic, she was all but forgotten. It's a cautionary tale for anyone who relies too heavily on only one aspect of the BQ to increase her appeal. You need to treat the whole package!

1930s—Katharine Hepburn

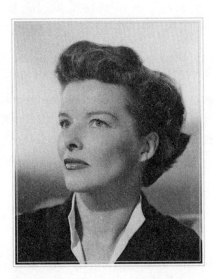

Katharine Hepburn had what was considered a "masculine" look and wore pants at a time when most women didn't dream of slipping them on.

- Her forehead is large and square.

- Her eyes are far apart and small, with low eyebrows.

- Her cheekbones are so pronounced that her face becomes extremely angular.

- Her lips are thin.

Yet this Hepburn was full of vigor, didn't mind being seen doing all kinds of sports, and was famous for her cold showers, salty humor, long walks, unconventional relationships, and a vivid zest for life. Her confidence in herself and her appearance gave her a very high BQ.

1940s—Ingrid Bergman

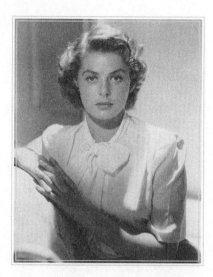

Ingrid Bergman went from being one of the most popular movie stars in the world to persona non grata in Hollywood when she left her husband to have an affair with a married film director, Roberto Rossellini, and bore his children. I think she was at her absolute most radiant when she fell in love with Rossellini. She just blossomed.

Ingrid always had an unusual beauty.

- Her face is very round, which is particularly notable as many actresses of her generation tended to have more sculpted faces.

- Her eyes are small, fairly close together, and heavy-lidded, becoming very crepey (crinkled and paperlike) as she grew older.

- Her nose has an unusual shape, with large nostrils.

- Her lower lip is much heavier than her upper lip, giving her a distinct pout.

- Her teeth are crooked.

Part of her high BQ comes from her unique ability to be both sexual and vulnerable, which is what has made the movie *Casablanca* such an enduring classic. She also displayed a stunningly high BQ in the film *Indiscreet*, made in 1958, when she was 43. In this romantic comedy, she played an actress opposite longtime friend Cary Grant, and her self-deprecating wit coupled with some of the most beautiful and figure-enhancing costumes ever created for her to wear on-screen were breathtaking. Watch it if you want to see what a "middle-aged" woman is capable of showing the world!

1950s—Audrey Hepburn

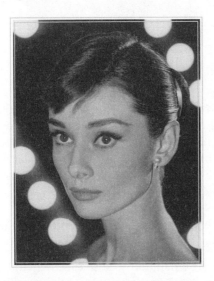

Audrey Hepburn's is one of my favorite faces of all time. I just cannot take my eyes off her. Yet when you deconstruct her face, you can see that her features, individually, are not always what you'd consider attractive.

- She has great bone structure, but her eyes are close together.

- Her eyebrows are enormous; very thick for the delicate proportions of the rest of her face.

- Her nose is slim but long.

- Her upper lip is small in proportion to her lower lip.

- Her lips are quite large in comparison to the size of her chin, which is small.

- She has a long, slender neck.

- Her body is extremely slim, verging on the way-too-skinny, and rather shapeless.

But somehow, when all placed together, these features made Audrey incandescently lovely, with a super-high BQ. She aged amazingly well. Had she lived longer, no doubt she would have remained one of the world's loveliest women.

1960s—Twiggy

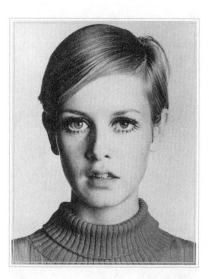

Love her or loathe her, Twiggy revolutionized fashion. She took some things that were huge deficits by the standards of beauty in the mid-1960s—a naturally super-skinny, bony, flat-chested body and knobby-kneed legs—and tweaked them to become one of history's more iconic women.

- Her forehead is high.

- She has beautiful big eyes that she soon learned to emphasize with deliberately large, fake eyelashes.

11

- She has a slim, nice nose.

- She has bony cheeks, because she had no fat on her face—
  they just stuck out!

- Her lips are a very unusual shape.

- She has a fairly small chin.

When Twiggy's hair was famously cut by Vidal Sassoon, her BQ went crazy. She found her look—and what a look it was. Compare Twiggy's androgynous, geometric look with the more curvy, flowing styles that had preceded her, and there was just no turning back. She became the definitive marker between old and mod.

1970s—Bette Midler

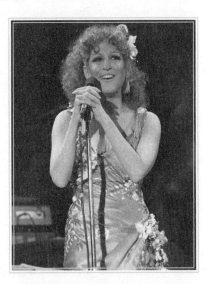

Bette Midler is a supremely gifted singer/actress, but her looks are far from what is considered classic. In fact, there's a French phrase to describe her iconic beauty: *jolie laide* literally means "pretty/ugly." However, due to her delicious personality, she positively radiates a fabulously sassy attitude as well as congeniality, which up her BQ remarkably. And as soon as she opens her mouth to sing, I just melt!

- Her forehead is unusually high and her face shape quite
  oval, so her cheekbones lack definition.

- Her hair can be a mess of frizz.

- Her eyes are hooded and small.

- Her nose is, well, distinctive.

- Her lips are large and saucy.

- Her chin is slightly receding.

1980s—Tina Turner

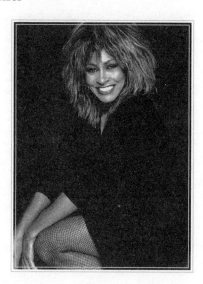

Talk about aging well. Tina Turner looked better when her comeback hit "What's Love Got to Do with It" went global in 1984 than she did as a star in 1960s. At the time, she was the oldest singer (age 45) in history to have a number-one hit, and boy, did her BQ go through the roof along with her record sales!

Tina was never considered a great beauty, but I'd call her stunning. Plus she's always had indefatigable energy, charisma, and the best legs in the business—she's the whole package.

- When she was younger, she wore hairstyles and heavy makeup that emphasized her already long and narrow face shape.

- Her eyes are piercing but small.

- Her nose is wide.

- Her chin is too small for the overall proportion of her face.

Which just goes to show that anyone can reinvent herself, no matter her age. There's nothing like a shot of confidence to improve your BQ!

1990s—Kate Moss

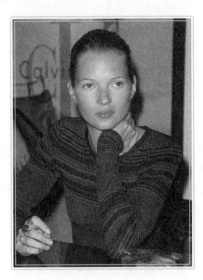

Okay, I must confess that Kate Moss is not my cup of tea, but obviously lots of people disagree with me as she's become one of the most successful models of all time. Kate's beauty is definitely not classic.

- She has a large forehead.

- Her eyes are small and set far apart.

- She has a small nose.

- She has prominent, bony cheeks.

- Her mouth has a funny sort of pucker.

- She has crummy teeth.

Still, I must also admit that Kate does have one of those super-idiosyncratic faces, and she has deftly parlayed her flaws into a career of fame and fortune.

2000s—Michelle Yeoh

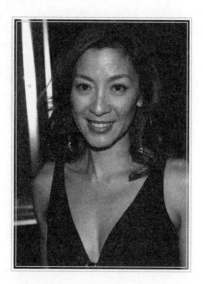

Named as one of *People* magazine's 50 Most Beautiful People in the World in 1997, after her role as a James Bond girl in *Tomorrow Never Dies*, Michelle Yeoh truly came into her beauty when she starred in the Academy Award–winning film, *Crouching Tiger, Hidden Dragon*, in 2000 at the age of 38. I think this feat was even more remarkable, as her female costar in that film was the lovely and much younger Ziyi Zhang. But I felt that Michelle's mature beauty was much sexier and subtle.

- Her face is round.
- Her eyes are large, extremely expressive, and almond-shaped with very little eyelid, as is typical for Asian women.
- Her nose is fairly wide, but it fits her face.
- Her mouth is not exceptional.
- She has a long, elegant neck.

15

Michelle has great sex appeal, which I believe is due in part to the self-confidence she has earned after her many years of determined training in martial arts. I think she's a knockout.

Once you see how these women enhanced their uniqueness, enabling their BQ to score into the stratosphere, you'll be better able to deconstruct other faces and personalities, including your own, so you can assess your strengths, as well as your weaknesses. In Part III, I'll show you how to use their techniques to enhance your own BQ—and you'll soon be convinced that recognizing and accentuating *your* positives are as important as improving your negatives.

CHAPTER TWO

The BQ Formula
10 Commandments

The BQ Formula program is about recognizing your inner and outer beauty, about changing your attitude, about being able to take an honest look at yourself. It's all about changing for the better, learning to analyze your good points and your bad points so that you can then devise a realistic plan to improve your appearance.

It's also about regaining your sense of self so you can effortlessly radiate confidence, competence, contentment, and charisma. Even when you are having a bad day, as long as you have self-confidence—in your abilities as well as with your appearance—you'll be able to cope with whatever life throws at you.

The BQ 10 Commandments are the foundation of the BQ Formula approach to beauty. They cover all the major points of this program, each hitting home in a different way. As soon as you start incorporating these commandments into your daily routine, your BQ will immediately go way up, because you'll automatically become more confident with your new attitude toward your own beauty. Refer back to these commandments whenever you have any questions or if your convictions start to waver.

BQ 1: OWN YOUR BEAUTY

Faye Dunaway once said that "the best thing for beauty is just being happy." You can be the most gorgeous woman in the world, but if you're down on yourself you won't look wonderful.

Owning your beauty means you accept and recognize the beautiful traits that you already possess. It also means that you build upon that foundation by enhancing and maximizing your best features *first*. Only after you've done that do you move on to tackling your weaknesses.

One of my colleagues, an anesthesiologist with an exceptionally beautiful, long, sculpted neck, came over to me one day and said, "I'm thinking about having my breasts done."

I looked at her in shock. "I hope you haven't caught me staring at you," I told her, "but you've got the most magnificent neck I've ever seen." She looked at me as if I'd grown two heads, but then quickly realized what I was saying. She gave me a swift hug and confessed that she knew she'd become fixated on her breasts and that maybe she was obsessing about the wrong thing. And guess what—she ended up not doing her breasts, after all.

It's easy to spot women who own their beauty. They're the smiling ones striding down the beach, clad in a bikini while proudly showing off their curves (while you might be wrapping a sarong around your behind the instant you get up, lest someone judge the tiny pooch of cellulite on your thighs). They're the ones walking down the street with their heads up, their backs straight, their clothing fitting them impeccably, and that je ne sais quoi, which is French for "I don't know what"—but is really a way to say, "That woman looks great, and I'm not sure what precisely she's done, but she's done it!"

You can't own your beauty if you aren't confident in your own skin.

BQ 2: ACCEPT YOUR GENETIC DESTINY . . . AND BUILD ON IT

I don't care how good a plastic surgeon is, if you love Megan Fox's nose but it's the wrong size and shape to fit properly with the rest of your face, you'll look terrible with it. Any surgeon who tells you otherwise is doing you a huge disservice.

Genetic destiny has brought many patients into my office. They're the ones who say, "I have my mother's hips." Or, "I have my father's nose." They might be good candidates for surgery if their father's nose is as large as Cyrano de Bergerac's, but they may also want to consider how much of their inherited appearance actually makes them uniquely beautiful.

Accepting your genetic destiny means you acknowledge your body type and height; the intrinsic shape of your face; and your predisposition to have broad shoulders like your father and wide hips like your mother. If you're five feet two, you're never going to be five foot ten; if you have a small bone structure, you're never going to be Angelina Jolie (and getting your lips plumped up will not make you look more like her). So there has to be a healthy amount of self-analysis as well as realistic expectations about the genetic factors affecting your BQ, and what surgery and other procedures can do for you.

Assess your strong points. Find your best features. Then be thrilled about them—and accentuate them to show them off in all their glory. You can't say it shouldn't be this or that or wish you were someone else. Be happy being you.

BQ 3: ACCEPT THE AGE YOU ARE . . .
AND MAKE IT BETTER

A woman came to me recently and said, "I'm sixty and I'm miserable about it."

I said, "Honey, you *are* sixty. What's your alternative? Your alternative is *dead*."

She had the good grace to smile and look a little sheepish. "Well, you do have a point," she admitted.

I smiled back. "Another way to think about getting older is to remember how many loved ones you might have lost when they were way too young," I replied. "Think about what they've missed—time with friends and family, seeing their children grow older, savoring all of life's pleasures and pains. *You* didn't miss any of that because *you* are still here!"

Sure, as we get older, it's hard to *not* think about the what-ifs, and I-wish-I-hads, but it's much healthier not to look to the past; you must live in the present to fully experience life at its best. So, whether you just change that recording in your head, or simply take a few minutes to close your eyes, take a deep breath, and start again, make mindfulness about everything that's made you be *you* (including your age and experience) a regular part of your daily routine.

The cliché that you're only as old as you feel is certainly true. Growing up, we had a family friend, an older gentleman who was like an adopted grandfather to me, who was quite short, with big blue eyes that gave him a sort of elfin quality. One day, when I was about 16, he took me golfing, and he deliberately swerved the cart around, as if to drive into the bushes. It would have been typical teenage behavior—except he was in his sixties at the time. I looked at him and said, "Just when are you gonna grow up?" Oh, he laughed and laughed.

His zest for life gave him an exceptionally high BQ. The merry twinkle in his eyes drew people to him until the day he died, when he was 82. He was a real touchstone for me of how an adult can accept his age—and run with it!

BQ 4: STOP WHINING, START DOING

Yep, this is the no-nonsense Commandment (which I'll cover in much greater detail in Part III). But taking the leap to incorporate changes into your life is one of the most important aspects of your BQ—because it covers the areas where you *can* control your own beauty.

Change is really hard. It's scary. And a lot of times it's a long journey until you reach that tipping point where you think, *Okay I can't stand it anymore,* and you finally get motivated to do what you know you need to do. That's when you start exercising, eating better, wearing sunscreen, sleeping more, and managing the stress and other frustrations in your life.

Best advice: Start small and work your way up. Have realistic expectations so you don't undermine yourself before you start.

BQ 5: THERE'S NO SUCH THING AS A PERMANENT QUICK FIX

I have no doubt that you've gone on some kind of fad diet at some point in your life. If you have, you know there is no magic pill or quick fix (like liposuction, as so many of my patients erroneously believe) that's going to get the weight off. It takes work and time to shed those pounds. It takes even more work to keep them off.

BQ is not just a concept—it's a life process. It's not a quick fix. It's not a fad diet or trendy skin-care regimen or lose-inches-instantly exercise routine. Although trendy diets or extreme exercise programs might get some weight off quickly, it will all come back unless you incorporate regular healthy eating and regular amounts of movement into your daily routine.

Improving your BQ is going to take some effort. But not difficult effort—*enjoyable* effort that will give you satisfying results as soon as you start the program. As you'll see once you go to Chapter 3 and calculate your BQ score that improving your BQ is done on your own time. You set the schedule. You make changes as you need to make them. There is no perfect score, and there is no deadline.

BQ 6: MAJOR CHANGES = MAJOR INVESTMENT (TIME, EMOTION, MONEY)

Most of the changes you make in your quest for a higher BQ will be deeply satisfying—which will certainly help motivate you—but you also need to remember that major changes don't come from minor tweaks. Sure, you can lose a few pounds if you stop drinking soda or alcohol, but you won't lose substantial weight unless you're willing to overhaul the way you eat. You won't make enormous changes in your wardrobe unless you're willing to make a blunt assessment of the clothes you already have hanging in your closet. You won't be happy with the nose job you've wanted to have for 30 years if you think it will make your unhappy marriage better.

As you know, anything worth doing is worth doing well. Only you can find the time and effort to make the commitment needed for the kind of lifestyle changes that will bring you lasting happiness. It is possible to create—and live with—an entirely new mind-set, no matter what your age. A mind-set that encompasses the big picture over your entire life—not a quick fix that you know will never last.

BQ 7: DON'T COMPARE YOURSELF TO OTHERS

Sure, Angelina Jolie has unusually big lips, but what she might not know is women with lips her size often will develop deeply etched nasolabial lines (running from the nose to the lips). How prominently these folds will appear is determined by genetics, but they start to become more noticeable when most women are in their forties.

The point is: everybody is unique. Some women have pert noses and some have huge honkers. Some heal really well after an injury or surgery, and some people have poor scarring or complications. Some burn every time they go in the sun and others get a creamy, golden tan. Some eat like pigs and never gain an ounce, while you just look at a piece of chocolate and it magically appears on your butt.

Comparing yourself to anyone else is an exercise in futility—it will only erode your self-confidence. Be happy with who you are and you'll instantly look happier and better!

BQ 8: DON'T GET STUCK IN A BEAUTY RUT

Beauty changes just like everything else in life. You're certainly not living and behaving as you did decades earlier, so why would you want to look the same way at 50 as you did at 20? Your beauty should evolve with you so it suits your personality, budget, and body type for your current stage of life. Those stuck in a beauty rut are unable to realistically assess their beauty while clinging to the same hairstyle, hair color, skin-care regimen, makeup, and clothing that no longer suit them.

You'll learn how to get out of your beauty rut as you read this book. I can't begin to tell you how liberating and fun it can be to finally trash your old makeup and learn new techniques to enhance your natural beauty (see Chapter 6 for that information). Finding your best look is an inherent part of raising your BQ.

BQ 9: STREAMLINE YOUR BEAUTY ROUTINE

Create a simple beauty routine that works for you, so you can dedicate yourself to doing it every day. With a routine that you know well and that you know makes you look great, you'll easily be able to look your best whenever you leave the house. Plus once you get the basics down and know what suits you best, you'll waste far less money buying makeup or clothing you'll never wear.

BQ 10: COUNT YOUR BLESSINGS

One of my patients was a young single mother, a gorgeous, vivacious redhead who came to me after a breast cancer diagnosis. Her reconstruction went well, and, like many of my breast cancer patients, she was happy not to have to see me again.

Fast-forward a few years, to one of those days when I was doing rounds in the hospital and feeling particularly sorry for myself because I was going bald. As I was walking toward the elevator, moping about my lost locks (that were, in my estimation, greatly lowering my BQ score), I heard a faint voice calling my name.

It was the same patient, although it took me a few seconds to recognize her. The cancer had returned, she barely weighed 90 pounds . . . and she was totally bald. Her gorgeous red hair had fallen out after chemotherapy, and she was a shadow of her former, energetic self.

She died several days later.

I walked out of there so angry at myself for moping about my hair. I had my health. I had my career. I had everything to live for—and so had she.

I'd like to tell this story to some of my patients who are obsessing about a tiny wrinkle only they can see. These patients don't really need a surgeon—they need some perspective!

I always think about the lovely redhead when I'm starting to feel sorry for myself. I can't justify throwing myself any pity parties when I have so many patients who need breast reconstruction or other noncosmetic surgical procedures because they are confronting life-threatening illnesses.

Like many who work in medicine, I don't take my good health for granted. I look at the big picture. I made it to age 54 with many professional accomplishments and a wonderful family that make me happy. When I hit the big 5-0 I heaved a sigh of relief that I didn't get testicular cancer or lymphoma or Hodgkin's disease or some other illness that tends to strike when you're younger.

Drawing up a list of the blessings you have is a wonderful exercise. For one thing, acknowledging all that has been good in your life is emotionally satisfying. For another, it will help you pinpoint what blessings you may wish to have more of—but know you have to work a little bit harder at getting.

Read on . . . I'll show you how true beauty is so much more than the wrinkles on your brow or the width of your nose; it is created as you live your life, express your feelings, and present yourself full of healthy, vibrant self-expression and self-worth.

PART II

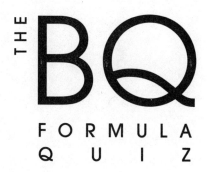

THE **BQ** FORMULA QUIZ

CHAPTER THREE

The BQ Formula Quiz

Think of your BQ score as a sort of lifestyle surgeon—without a scalpel!

After answering all the questions, you will be given your own BQ score. It will tell you where your strengths and weaknesses lie, and will help you identify areas that need improvement—whether in your beauty regimen, exercise, clothing style, genetic destiny, or a combination.

Once you know your score, you can go first to the appropriate section of this book for treatments and advice about how to raise your BQ.

I. GENETIC DESTINY

Genetic destiny refers to the features that you've inherited, such as the shape of your face, features, and body. These cannot be changed without treatment from a qualified MD or surgeon.

1. *What is your ethnicity?*
   A. Black
   B. Asian
   C. Caucasian
   D. Hispanic/Latino
   E. Mixed race

2. **What is your skin type?**
   A. Type I or Type II (extremely fair to fair skin—tendency to freckles and burns)
   B. Type III (medium skin—sometimes burns and often tans)
   C. Type IV (olive skin—rarely burns and easily tans)
   D. Type V or Type VI (dark brown to black skin—very rarely burns)

3. **What is your body shape?**
   A. Hourglass
   B. Apple
   C. Pear
   D. String bean

4. **What is your tendency to put on muscle?**
   A. I'm a mesomorph (I put on muscle easily)
   B. I'm an ectomorph (I'm lean and don't muscle easily)
   C. I'm an endomorph (I tend to be round and soft)
   D. I'm a combination

5. **How dry or oily is your skin?**
   A. Oily but clear
   B. Oily with adult acne (so unfair!)
   C. Dry
   D. Very dry
   E. Normal

6. **How many wrinkles do you have?**
   A. A few around my eyes and on my forehead
   B. Some, but they're age appropriate
   C. Too many, and I'm very unhappy about it
   D. The fine wrinkles don't bother me, but I really don't like the deeper grooves near my nose and on my forehead

7. **Are your eyes your most striking feature?**
   A. Yes
   B. No, they're too small for my face
   C. No, they're too close together
   D. No, they're heavy-lidded, so I always look tired
   E. No, they are not the most striking feature, but they are attractive

8. Do you have bags under your eyes?
   A. My parents have bags, but I don't yet
   B. Yes, and I hate them
   C. I'm getting older, and I'm just starting to notice them
   D. They're barely noticeable
   E. No, and my parents' eyes have aged nicely

9. How would you describe your forehead?
   A. Etched with deep grooves
   B. Just right
   C. Making my eyebrows droop
   D. Too prominent

10. My cheekbones are:
   A. Prominent
   B. Round and smooth
   C. Looking a little gaunt
   D. I don't have much definition in my cheeks anymore

11. Do you have a prominent nasolabial fold (the lines between your nose and lips that form when you smile)?
   A. Yes, deeply grooved
   B. Yes, but it's not very deep
   C. My skin is still smooth
   D. My parents do, so I expect mine to show up any day now
   E. I have a big smile, so my grooves are prominent, but my smile makes up for it

12. How would you describe your nose?
   A. Too small
   B. Too big—thanks a whole lot, Mom and Dad!
   C. Too wide
   D. Crooked—I broke it while playing sports
   E. Fits my face

13. My lips are:
   A. As big as Angelina's, and they're all mine
   B. Too small
   C. Getting thinner with age
   D. Not perfect, but I like them

14. How would you describe your neck?
A. Driving me crazy with those weird bands sticking out
B. Crepey
C. Smooth and firm
D. Drooping and/or fatty
E. Long
F. Short and thick

15. My décolleté (low neckline) is:
A. Smooth and clear
B. A bit freckled and mottled
C. Getting crepey and looking blah
D. So unattractive I now prefer to cover it up

16. How would you describe your hair?
A. Thin
B. Thinning
C. Curly
D. Thick
E. Average but rich and shiny, because I take care of it

17. My breasts are:
A. Too big
B. Too small
C. Sagging naturally, or from breastfeeding or weight loss
D. Just right, with the size and shape proportional to my body

18. How would you describe your midsection?
A. Too flabby but I never exercise
B. Too flabby even though I do zillions of crunches
C. Too flabby after childbirth
D. Firm and defined—I earned that six pack!
E. Flat but not firm

19. My buttocks and upper legs are:
A. Too flabby but I never exercise
B. Too flabby even though I do zillions of squats
C. I have cellulite and nothing gets rid of it
D. Nice and smooth—I earned my perky butt!
E. Thin, but not firm

20. How would you describe your hands?
A. Smooth and clear
B. Getting a lot of freckles
C. Looking kind of veiny and thin-skinned
D. Giving my age away
E. Looking fine because I take care of my nails with regular manicures (at home or at a salon)

21. I have been told I look like:
A. A famous movie or TV star
B. A famous athlete
C. A famous model
D. None of the above, but I possess traits of each of above
E. Nobody famous, just me, and I'm OK with that

22. My best feature is:
A. Nothing major
B. One aspect of my face
C. One aspect of my breasts
D. One aspect of my body
E. More than one aspect of my body or face

23. My worst feature is:
A. Nothing major
B. One aspect of my face
C. One aspect of my breasts
D. One aspect of my body
E. More than one aspect of my body or face

24. Are you comfortable highlighting your best feature and down-playing your worst?
A. Absolutely—then I know I'm looking my best.
B. Sometimes—for example, I know I need to wear more makeup than usual to play up my eyes, so I save it for special occasions
C. I'd like to, but I don't know how
D. I don't want to think about my best or worst features

II. CURRENT HABITS

Your current habits apply to your physical and mental health. These factors of your BQ are entirely under your control.

Self-image

25. Are you basically happy with your life?
- A. No
- B. Yes
- C. Sometimes
- D. I don't know how to answer this question—it scares me

26. Are you confident about your appearance?
- A. No
- B. Yes
- C. Sometimes
- D. I don't think I'll ever figure it out

27. Are you confident about life in general?
- A. No
- B. Yes
- C. Sometimes
- D. I lose sleep at night from the anxious worrying about my future

28. When it comes to self-image, how do you deal with your insecurities and fears?
- A. Talk to friends and loved ones
- B. See a therapist, who really helps me understand myself
- C. I don't deal with them very well
- D. A nice glass of wine helps
- E. Bluster my way through in public, then collapse in private

29. Do you believe you think about your image a little too much?
- A. Okay, so maybe I have a few too many mirrors, but so does everyone else I know
- B. I don't think about it enough!
- C. Only if I have an important event to go to that takes me out of my comfort zone
- D. Not really—I like how I look

30. **What is your opinion of those who seem obsessed with their appearance?**
  A. They're so shallow and deluded!
  B. I feel sorry for anyone who's so consumed by the surface of things
  C. It's their life—they can do what they want!
  D. I'm glad it isn't me, as I've got more important things to worry about

31. **Do you find it hard to get motivated to make needed changes in your life?**
  A. Yes
  B. No
  C. It depends on the situation
  D. I find it hard to start, but once I do, I'm tenacious

32. **Do you tend to binge (food, drink, behavior) as a form of self-comfort?**
  A. Yes
  B. No
  C. Sometimes
  D. Often (more than once a month)

33. **Are you married or in a satisfying relationship?**
  A. Yes
  B. No
  C. I'm not in a relationship but am satisfied with my life right now
  D. Not being in a satisfying relationship right now is causing depression or anxiety

34. **Do the people in your life compliment you and make you feel good about yourself and the way you look?**
  A. Yes
  B. No
  C. Sometimes
  D. Never

Skin Care

35. Do you use a moisturizer as per your skin's needs?
A. Always
B. When I remember to—it's not that important
C. I have oily skin, so I don't think I need a moisturizer
D. Never

36. Do you have a skin-care regimen?
A. Yes, but I don't remember to do it all the time
B. No, because nothing I've tried seems to make a difference
C. Yes, and I do it religiously every day
D. Sort of, because I'm fickle about products and change my regimen often

37. Do you constantly change your skin-care products?
A. I've used the same stuff for the last ten years—it works, so why bother changing?
B. Yes, because when I don't see results quickly, I need to try something new
C. I give my products at least six to eight weeks of regular use before changing
D. It doesn't really matter what I use—it's all hype, anyway

38. Do you clean your face and remove your makeup at night?
A. When I remember to
B. Scrupulously, every night, no matter what
C. Yes, but I use my baby's wipes as I'm really pooped
D. It's no big deal to do it in the morning, if I've forgotten

39. If you have problem skin, what do you do?
A. Listen to recommendations from the women at the cosmetics counters
B. Listen to the recommendations of my facialist
C. Go to a dermatologist
D. Self-treat and get advice from Websites or magazines

Sleep

40. Do you get a minimum of seven to eight hours of uninterrupted, deep sleep at night?
   A. I try to, at least once or twice during the week and on weekends
   B. I always do—I can't function without a good night's sleep
   C. I catch up on weekends
   D. Never

41. When you do get to sleep, is your sleep restful and refreshing?
   A. Always
   B Most of the time
   C. Sometimes
   D. Not enough
   E. Almost never

Exercise

42. How often do you engage in a good cardiovascular exercise routine?
   A. Three to five times per week
   B. Two to three times per week
   C. Once in a while, if I feel like it or have recently eaten too much
   D. When I remember, and then I work out extra-hard
   E. Never

43. Do you engage in a weight-training program?
   A. Yes, regularly
   B. No, never
   C. Sometimes, if I'm in the gym and see other women doing it
   D. When I remember, but I don't think I'm doing it right

44. Do you try to mix up your exercise routine?
   A. Once in a while
   B. Yes, otherwise I get bored
   C. Never
   D. I wonder if I'm too fickle; I have a hard time sticking to anything

45. Do you work out even when you don't really want to?
   A. Yes, for the stress relief and other benefits
   B. Sometimes, as I really have a super-busy life
   C. Once in a while, just so I don't feel guilty
   D. I know I should, but I don't

46. Are you conscious about your posture?
   A. I tend to slump, but it's no big deal
   B. I really do sit and stand straight as much as I possibly can
   C. It's not something I think about
   D. I straighten up only when I realize my back is hurting
   E. My posture is great because I work my core muscles and am aware of my posture at all times

47. How would you describe the way you walk?
   A. Like a model sashaying down the catwalk
   B. Long slow strides
   C. Short quick steps
   D. Irregular steps, depending if I am late for an appointment
   E. I have never noticed

Smoking

48. Do you smoke?
   A. Only when I go out at night—occasionally
   B. Never
   C. Less than a pack a day
   D. More than a pack a day

49. What happened when you tried to quit smoking?
   A. I quit easily and haven't smoked since!
   B. I've tried every possible method, and now I smoke more than ever
   C. I've cut down from one or more packs to just a few cigarettes every day
   D. I still sneak a few cigarettes now and then but can keep the urge under control
   E. Every time I try to quit, I gain weight, so I go back to smoking
   F. I finally quit but gained weight that I cannot lose
   G. I have never smoked

Stress

50. How do you manage your stress?
A. I don't manage it; it manages me
B. Yoga, meditation, mindful breathing
C. I talk someone or spend time on a favorite hobby
D. Screaming into a pillow
E. All, or nearly all of the above

51. People who know me best would say that I handle stress in one of the following ways:
A. Very well—I recognize the situation and deal rationally with it
B. Fairly well, but there is room for improvement
C. Inconsistently—sometimes well, sometimes I lose it
D. Poorly—when the wrong buttons are pressed, I lose control

52. After a stressful situation, which of the following occurs:
A. I calm down immediately after using my favorite stress-busting technique
B. I calm down after a while
C. I eventually calm down, but it takes a while and I may have said or done something stupid
D. I calm down after I kick or throw something, yell, or have a long cry
E. I don't handle stress well, and I don't know what to do about it

Sun Exposure

53. How often do you go in the sun?
A. I avoid it like the plague
B. Just normal outside exposure
C. I like how the sun feels, and having a tan makes me look better
D. Donatella Versace is my role model—I can't be baked enough!
E. I like the outdoors, but I use sunscreen appropriately

54. When you do go outside, do you wear sunscreen?
  A. Every day; it's as important as brushing my teeth
  B. In the summertime when it's really hot and I remember
  C. On vacation so I don't get fried
  D. I don't believe in sunscreen—a nice tan makes me feel and look younger
  E. When I play outdoors, I use it, but not during the workweek

Nutrition

55. Is eating a diet that you know is as healthy as possible (whole grains, limited protein, good fats, lots of fruits and vegetables, minimal sugar) one of your top priorities?
  A. Not enough
  B. Always
  C. Most of the time
  D. I really need to stop eating so much junk food, but I need help

56. How often do you eat nourishing home-cooked meals?
  A. Most of the time as healthful as possible
  B. Always (unless I'm going out for a meal)—I need to know everything about what's going in my mouth!
  C. I try to, when I have the time
  D. Once in a long while

57. Do you take supplements?
  A. A good multivitamin-and-mineral supplement with calcium
  B. I take so many supplements I can't see the counter
  C. When I remember
  D. Never

58. How much alcohol do you drink, and what kind of alcohol is it?
  A. Maybe one drink four to seven nights a week
  B. I never drink
  C. I drink socially—a few drinks at least once a week
  D. I think I might be drinking a little bit too much

III. STYLE

And finally, style—clothing, accessories, makeup, and hair. These factors are purely physical and totally under your control. Your BQ can increase or decrease based on what you do with these elements.

59. What philosophy best describes you regarding your wardrobe?
   A. I dress conservatively because it is safe
   B. I have great legs and wear elegant dresses and skirts to bare them as often as possible
   C. I have nice cleavage but wear lots of sweaters and scarves because I'm pretty shy
   D. I have nice cleavage and, when appropriate, I show it proudly
   E. I try to hide as many flaws as possible with my wardrobe

60. Do you have what you consider to be a signature style?
   A. Yes, and it saves me a ton of time getting dressed in the morning
   B. I want to have one, but I don't know where to start
   C. For certain occasions, yes, so I'm inconsistent
   D. Style is not one of my priorities

61. Is it easy for you to make up your mind when you go shopping for new clothes?
   A. Yes
   B. No
   C. Most of the time
   D. Never, and I'm always returning things after I buy them, too
   E. Too easy—my credit card debt is getting scary

62. Do you have certain outfits that fit you well and that you know make you look great?
   A. I have some casual outfits I like, but nothing dressy
   B. Yes—I'm pretty confident about my style and dress to enhance it
   C. I know I need to take my clothes to the tailor so they fit better
   D. I think I need style help but don't know where to go to get it
   E. I'm not thinking about my wardrobe until I lose 20 pounds

63. Do you feel that you dress appropriately for your age?
   A. Yes, always
   B. Most of the time
   C. Sometimes yes, sometimes no—it depends on the occasion
   D. I know I should stop wearing my daughter's jeans

64. Is your closet full of clothes you never wear?
   A. Yes—I'm a pack rat
   B. Yes, because my weight fluctuates so I have lots of different sizes
   C. Not at all; I revamp my wardrobe every season
   D. I keep some old clothes for sentimental reasons

65. Do you ever wear shoes or boots that look great but hurt your feet or body?
   A. Never—I value my feet too much
   B. Only for special occasions and for a very short period, and then I change into something more comfortable
   C. I wear high heels more than I should, but I draw the line at real pain
   D. Pain is irrelevant if the shoes are to die for!

66. Are you happy with your wardrobe of accessories, and do you wear them often?
   A. Yes, and they're so much fun to play around with
   B. I only have a few key pieces, but they're more than adequate for my look
   C. Accessories are overrated!
   D. I'd like to get some, but I need advice
   E. I'm strictly a casual kind of person, so accessorizing is never going to be a priority

67. Do you have a signature piece of jewelry?
   A. One piece only
   B. I don't like jewelry
   C. I'd like to, but I can't afford expensive jewelry
   D. I have an incredible selection of jewelry, and never get tired of wearing it
   E. I envy people who can wear jewelry with ease. I don't like people looking at me when I wear something flashy

68. *If I need vision correction, I:*
  A. Don't need correction, or I wear contacts
  B. Hate wearing glasses; they remind me of being taunted as a kid
  C. Are not crazy about them but I'm resigned to having to wear them
  D. Collect and flaunt my fabulous glasses collection, since they are as important an accessory as shoes and handbag
  E. Look great in glasses, and like the change in appearance that they bring

69. *Who do you dress to please?*
  A. Myself
  B. My husband/partner (if applicable, and if their taste is reasonable!)
  C. My friends
  D. My colleagues at work, as we have a fairly strict dress code
  E. I don't really think much about clothes

70. *Do you update your hairstyle?*
  A. I think I might want to do something but don't know where to start
  B. All the time—my hair is as important to my appearance as my clothing
  C. I am too scared to cut my hair; it's like a security blanket for me
  D. Never—I like it the way it is, and so does my family

71. *Does your hairstyle work with your facial structure?*
  A. Yes, I know it does
  B. My hairstylist says it does, but I'm not so sure
  C. I never really thought about it
  D. I know I need to do something, because my face has changed over the years

72. Do you color your hair?
  A. Yes, I need to, as my roots are really obvious and very aging
  B. I don't need to (yet!)
  C. I am going gray, but it doesn't bother me
  D. No, my hair has gone totally gray or white, and I like it
  E. I highlight my hair when I want a new look
  F. Yes, I do it myself, and I use whatever is on sale at the drugstore

73. Are you happy with the shape of your eyebrows?
  A. Yes, they're just right for my face
  B. I overtweezed them, so they're too thin
  C. I don't pay any attention to my eyebrows
  D. I never seem to get them quite right

74. Do you have a makeup routine that you're happy with?
  A. Yes—I know what colors suit me, and I've got the application down to a science
  B. I'm good at doing casual makeup, but nothing more
  C. I don't believe in wearing makeup
  D. I haven't changed my makeup routine since I was a teenager
  E. I let the department store makeup ladies convince me what looks good

75. Do you know a lot of makeup tricks to enhance your appearance?
  A. I don't wear makeup
  B. Yes, I'm always looking for new ideas
  C. I stick to the tried and true
  D. Occasionally, if I have a special event to go to

ANSWER KEY FOR THE BQ QUIZ

Each question has a mathematically weighted answer. In the charts below, total your scores for each section.

BQ Quiz Part I Scoring							
1.	A = 4 B = 4 C = 4 D = 4 E = 4	2.	A = 0 B = 4 C = 6 D = 7	3.	A = 5 B = 4 C = 4 D = 5	4.	A = 6 B = 6 C = 1 D = 7
5.	A = 6 B = 4 C = 4 D = 0 E = 6	6.	A = 5 B = 5 C = 2 D = 4	7.	A = 7 B = 1 C = 1 D = 1 E = 6	8.	A = 5 B = 2 C = 2 D = 5 E = 5
9.	A = 0 B = 5 C = 0 D = 2	10.	A = 5 B = 5 C = 2 D = 2	11.	A = 0 B = 4 C = 5 D = 5 E = 5	12.	A = 5 B = 2 C = 2 D = -1 E = 5
13.	A = 6 B = 1 C = 1 D = 7	14.	A = 0 B = 0 C = 6 D = -1 E = 6 F = 2	15.	A = 7 B = 1 C = 0 D = 0	16.	A = 4 B = 1 C = 6 D = 6 E = 7
17.	A = 4 B = 4 C = 4 D = 5	18.	A = -4 B = -2 C = 0 D = 12 E = 7	19.	A = 3 B = 1 C = -1 D = 10 E = 6	20.	A = 5 B = 3 C = 2 D = 0 E = 4
21.	A = 5 B = 5 C = 5 D = 6 E = 6	22.	A = 1 B = 6 C = 6 D = 6 E = 8	23.	A = 9 B = 1 C = 1 D = -2 E = -4	24.	A = 12 B = 7 C = 0 D = -5
Total:							

BQ Quiz Part II Scoring							
25.	A = 1 B = 5 C = 3 D = 2	26.	A = 0 B = 6 C = 1 D = -1	27.	A = -1 B = 6 C = 0 D = -2	28.	A = 5 B = 5 C = -1 D = 0 E = -2
29.	A = 1 B = 1 C = 2 D = 5	30.	A = 3 B = 4 C = 3 D = 5	31.	A = -2 B = 4 C = 3 D = 5	32.	A = -2 B = 5 C = -1 D = -3
33.	A = 4 B = 3 C = 5 D = -1	34.	A = 4 B = 1 C = 3 D = 1	35.	A = 6 B = 4 C = 0 D = -2	36.	A = 0 B = -2 C = 6 D = 0
37.	A = 5 B = -2 C = 6 D = -1	38.	A = 0 B = 7 C = 0 D = -2	39.	A = 0 B = 2 C = 6 D = 0	40.	A = 4 B = 7 C = 0 D = -1
41.	A = 5 B = 4 C = 2 D = 0 E = -1	42.	A = 7 B = 6 C = -1 D = 0 E = -2	43.	A = 7 B = -2 C = -1 D = -1	44.	A = 5 B = 7 C = -1 D = -2
45.	A = 7 B = 5 C = -1 D = -2	46.	A = -2 B = 6 C = -2 D = -1 E = 7	47.	A = 6 B = 4 C = 1 D = -2 E = -2	48.	A = 0 B = 7 C = -1 D = -2
49.	A = 7 B = -2 C = -1 D = -1 E = -1 F = 5 G = 3	50.	A = -2 B = 7 C = 7 D = -1 E = 7	51.	A = 7 B = 5 C = -1 D = -2	52.	A = 7 B = 5 C = -1 D = -2 E = -2

53.	A = 7	54.	A = 7	55.	A = -1	56.	A = 6
	B = 4		B = -1		B = 7		B = 7
	C = -1		C = 0		C = 6		C = 4
	D = -2		D = -2		D = -2		D = -1
	E = 5		E = 1				
57.	A = 7	58.	A = 5				
	B = 4		B = 5				
	C = 4		C = 4				
	D = -1		D = 0				
Total:							

BQ Quiz Part III Scoring							
59.	A = -4	60.	A = 10	61.	A = 8	62.	A = 5
	B = 10		B = -1		B = -1		B = 7
	C = -1		C = 5		C = 5		C = 0
	D = 10		D = -4		D = -2		D = 0
	E = -4				E = -2		E = -1
63.	A = 10	64.	A = -4	65.	A = 7	66.	A = 10
	B = 5		B = -2		B = 4		B = 8
	C = -2		C = 10		C = 1		C = -3
	D = -4		D = 5		D = 1		D = -1
							E = -3
67.	A = 10	68.	A = 6	69.	A = 8	70.	A = -4
	B = -1		B = -4		B = 6		B = 10
	C = -2		C = 1		C = -2		C = -2
	D = 10		D = 10		D = 1		D = -2
	E = -1		E = 8		E = -4		
71.	A = 10	72.	A = 10	73.	A = 10	74.	A = 10
	B = 5		B = 6		B = -2		B = 5
	C = -4		C = 5		C = -4		C = -4
	D = -2		D = 6		D = -2		D = -4
			E = 8				E = 1
			F = -4				

75.	A = -4			
	B = 10			
	C = -1			
	D = 1			
Total:				

SCORING THE BQ FORMULA QUIZ

- The maximum score for Section I is 160. If you score less than 135 for questions 1–24, go to Appendices A, B, and C.

- The maximum score for Section II is 210. If you score less than 145 for questions 25–58, go to the following sections in the book:

Question Number	Topic	Page Number
25–34	Self-image	52
35–39	Skin care	78
40–41	Sleep	84
42–47	Exercise	87 and Appendix D
48–49	Smoking	93
50–52	Stress	71
53–54	Sun exposure	82
55–58	Nutrition	91

- The maximum score for Section III is 160. If you score less than 120 for questions 59–75, see the specific plans in Chapter 8 and refer to the following sections in Chapter 6:

Question Number	Topic	Page Number
59–69	Clothing	107
70–72	Hair	122
73–75	Makeup	127

When looking at your score and before you start working to improve your BQ, keep these basic principles in mind:

- There is no perfect BQ score.

- There is no "failing" the quiz. There are some areas that might need more work than others—that's all!

- Improving your BQ is a work in progress.

- You do *not* have to give something up to improve your BQ. Instead you should focus on this question: what do I have already that I can embrace and enhance?

- Don't compare yourself to anyone else. You are unique!

- Work at your own pace. This is not a race. Think of it as a journey. You are not competing with anyone.

- The quiz has been deliberately designed with several sections so that you can see your strengths and weaknesses in different areas. Don't be put off if you have a lot of numbers in Column 2—they're merely an indication of the areas you might want to tackle first.

- If you see that you might need to make changes in several different areas, don't worry. Instead of being overwhelmed, start with something small. Pick the area that you know you'll be able to do more easily *first*, because then you will have the satisfaction of making those changes and seeing results, thereby raising your score and giving you a boost of confidence. Then take the quiz again for only the section you've worked on, give yourself some much deserved acknowledgment and move on to another section.

- Trying to do too much at once is much harder than making small, incremental steps. This is not a quick-fix program— it's a program for life.

- After you've spent some time making the changes you'll learn about in the rest of the book, retake the quiz. When you want to do this is entirely up to you. Some quiz takers like to revisit their scores every month; others every three to six months, depending on their goals. There is no right or wrong—just what works for *you*. (Although, of course, it is extremely gratifying to revisit your initial quiz scores after you've made distinctive and noticeable changes in your appearance!)

- More than anything, the fact that you've taken the quiz and have decided to make some changes in your life has already raised your score!

So, now, let's begin! The chapters in Part III will show what you can do to get the highest BQ possible *without* the need for medical procedures or surgery. However, if you do decide on these procedures, more information can be found in the appendixes. Once your BQ score moves up, your confidence will get a huge boost, which will in turn then raise your score even higher.

PART III

HOW TO MAXIMIZE YOUR OWN

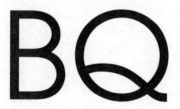

CHAPTER FOUR

Psychological Health

If you don't own your beauty, who will?

I can't tell you how many patients sit in my office, and when I give them a compliment about, say, their eyes, they'll say, "Really? My eyes? You're kidding! I think they look *horrible*." And then I know immediately that there's a self-image problem at play.

The key to the BQ Formula philosophy is to focus on the good points first, instead of fixating on the bad. So many of the beauty issues that we're dealing with have to do with denial and self-sacrifice (as in starving yourself to fit a misguided notion that ultra-thin equals ultra-beautiful) and unfair comparisons (especially to those friends or acquaintances who may have won the genetic lottery giving them a super-fast metabolism so they can eat what they want, or who have a perfectly proportioned nose when you do not).

In this chapter, I'm going to help you work on basics about self-esteem so you can then apply this new confidence to all other aspects of your appearance. You'll learn how accentuating the positive can only come after you turn off the negative tapes in your head, and that identifying and writing down your good points can help reinforce your feelings about them. Friends and loved ones can be used as a terrific barometer to gauge and improve attributes you might not even be aware of. There's also a Vanity vs. Narcissism Quiz to help you nurture healthy vanity and indentify the kind of narcissistic behavior that automatically reduces a BQ score.

HEALTHY VANITY VS. NARCISSISM

First, let me assure you that wanting to look the best you can and having a healthy self-esteem about your looks is *not* narcissism. It's what I call healthy vanity, and it's very important to having a high BQ. A certain amount of this healthy vanity is a good thing. It points to a high level of self-assurance and a level of comfort with yourself that is very attractive. People with a healthy vanity are able to see and work with their good and bad points to the best of their ability. They have a realistic and healthy view of themselves and others.

A narcissist, on the other hand, is someone obsessed with looks, status, or anything that can be lorded over others who are less fortunate. Narcissists are often notoriously unable to understand that their inflated views of themselves verge on the pathological, which means they need professional help to manage their grandiosity.

Taking the Healthy Vanity vs. Narcissism Quiz will show you how to identify which traits point to healthy vanity and which ones are indicative of an unhealthy self-absorption or narcissism. In my experience, narcissists usually are unaware of the extent of their fixation. If you have trouble identifying which of these traits is healthy vanity versus narcissism, or if the narcissistic traits apply to you, you may want to seek the help of a competent mental health professional. Narcissism is a psychological issue that should be addressed. It is, at the very least, a serious personality flaw, or, in worse cases, a recognized psychological disorder. Its antisocial aspects can have an extremely negative effect on a sufferer's daily life, personal relationships, and performance at work.

VANITY VS. NARCISSISM QUIZ

Answer each question with a V for Vanity or N for Narcissism. Scoring follows the quiz.

1. I care about how I look.   V   N

2. I'm usually late when I go out, because I know I'm going to make a sensational impression on everyone who sees me.
    V   N

3. I always judge people based on how they look.   V   N

4. It's natural to be worried about how you look, how you feel, and how you perform in our age-prejudiced world.   V   N

5. I'm turning 30, and if I get any wrinkles I'll go crazy.   V   N

6. I'm turning 40, and I want to minimize wrinkles.   V   N

7. I'm considering using injectible substances to help erase frown lines because they make me look tired and angry.   V   N

8. I love going to Botox parties every month or so—they're so much fun!   V   N

9. I know that plastic surgery will change my life.   V   N

10. If I'm out to dinner and there's a mirror in the restaurant, I look in it only to check to see if there's anything stuck in my teeth.   V   N

11. If I'm out to dinner and there's a mirror in the restaurant, I obsessively check myself because I know I look fabulous.   V   N

12. I can't look at myself without touching or rearranging my hair.   V   N

13. Sometimes I can't help myself from thinking, *I don't know what I would do if I weren't so good-looking.*   V   N

14. Once in a while, I can't help myself from thinking, *Wouldn't my life or career be so much better if I were prettier, even though I know deep down that I'd rather be judged on my brains and not my looks.*   V   N

15. I obsessively scan the women's magazines looking for the newest procedures, and I make an appointment as soon as I read about something that sounds great.   V   N

16. I always deny having had any cosmetic work done.   V   N

17. I have to admit that sometimes I like to hear gossip about who's had what done even though I know it isn't particularly nice.   V   N

18. I love to spread good gossip about who's had what cosmetic work done.   V   N

19. I can't help myself from being critical of my friends when they let themselves go, because, in my experience, people who let themselves go have stopped caring and their diminished self-esteem shows on the outside.   V   N

20. When I get to a restaurant and they don't give me the best table, I can't believe it. Everybody should be able to see how gorgeous I look.   V   N

21. I'm not thrilled about having to go to the gym after a long day, but I know I have to exercise to stay in shape, so I force myself to go anyway.   V   N

22. I need to know that I have the best figure of anyone else in the gym, or else I just want to cry.   V   N

23. I think anyone who is morbidly obese is lazy, and I don't care if that's a super-judgmental statement.   V   N

24. I make sure that the size tags are visible when I drape my coat over a chair at a restaurant, so everyone can see that I'm a size 0.   V   N

25. I'll go back to my plastic surgeon multiple times because that darn doctor just didn't get it right the first time, and I need to look perfect.   V   N

26. Some of the time, I look at myself and say, "You look pretty darn good today!"   V   N

27. I see defects in my face or visible body parts that no one else does.   V   N

28. The more procedures I have, the younger and more beautiful I'll look.   V   N

29. I'll do whatever it takes to be thin!   V   N

30. I may have stopped lying about my age once I hit 75, but my looks still matter!   V   N

Vanity vs. Narcissism Quiz Scoring					
1. V	2. N	3. N	4. V	5. N	6. V
7. V	8. N	9. N	10. V	11. N	12. N
13. N	14. V	15. N	16. N	17. V	18. N
19. V	20. N	21. V	22. N	23. N	24. N
25. N	26. V	27. N	28. N	29. N	30. V

After looking at the answers, you should have a pretty good idea of the traits of both healthy vanity and unhealthy narcissism. The goal of the BQ program is to help you have a realistic outlook on your looks and your life. That kind of self-knowledge and acceptance of the aging process will always raise your BQ score.

For example, when my mother was about to turn 90, she suddenly informed me that she wanted a face-lift! This lucid, stubborn, and usually healthily vain woman reminded me that she was in perfect health, requiring no heart, blood pressure, or other medications. She also reminded me that I was her son, and she asked little from me during my lifetime. (Talk about piling on the guilt!) I convinced her to let me apply a Botox treatment to her forehead, which raised her brow slightly and pleased her immensely. Her healthy vanity remained intact.

Healthy vanity, like my mother's, is at the heart of the BQ philosophy. You should be confident if you're good at something, and you should feel proud if you look good—that's normal. Doing something for attention (such as wearing provocative clothing), having a distorted image of yourself as you grow older (such as fixating on minuscule flaws), or expecting a plastic surgeon to "fix" your self-perceived problems without a willingness to address them yourself are all classic signs of narcissism.

Warning Signs of Narcissism and Appearance Obsession

Most plastic surgeons develop a sixth sense when talking to new patients. We size up the body language, how comfortable patients seem, how willing they are to discuss their hopes and fears, and how realistic their expectations are. Certain key phrases are giveaways that these patients might be better served by a competent therapist than a surgeon.

"I need this done. I have to have this procedure."

Whenever I hear that, I gently explain that cosmetic surgery is called elective for a reason. It's not necessary from a medical standpoint. No one will die without this procedure. At that point, I'm looking for more cues that a patient might be suffering from depression. Few come out and admit that they are. They might not list antidepressants on their medical form if they don't want me to know. So I'll try to steer our conversation toward acknowledging that depression might be an issue, and I make it clear that I won't operate on them unless they see a therapist first.

"I need a guarantee that I'm going to look like this."

I'll explain that cosmetic surgery (and medicine in general, for that matter), is not an exact science, and that everybody is different. Some people heal well after complicated surgery, and some don't. If patients still demand a guarantee, no matter what the procedure, then I'll just say that I can't help them.

"I only want a correction of 1.2 millimeters."

Anyone who has measured any part of their body down to a fraction may be suffering from *body dysmorphic disorder*, which is a fixation on perceived "deformities" that in reality are absolutely normal. Body dysmorphic disorder can become dangerous if not treated with therapy, as sufferers can continue to demand surgery and other procedures from less-than-ethical surgeons or physicians, to the point where the damage cannot be undone.

"I want to look young again, like when I was a teenager."

Having unrealistic expectations of what surgery can do to make you look younger is a typical warning sign of narcissism. It is also one of the most common comments I hear from patients who expect to erase decades from their appearance. Not only is this impossible, it is a warning sign to me that there are deep-seated psychological issues to address. Sure, we all want to turn the clock back a little, but expecting to look like a college freshman when your *granddaughter* is a college freshman is not going to happen!

I also notice this right away with someone who immediately talks about extremes, such as an especially petite woman who wants incredibly large breasts. She's likely to already have a high standard of self-esteem and knows she looks good. She just wants to do something to be noticed, not for her, but for an external quality. That's crossing over the line to narcissistic thinking.

NURTURING HEALTHY VANITY

Years ago I had a new patient who told me that he was a judge, and he took his job and the legal system very seriously. But the problem was he had a scowl on his face, and he looked perpetually angry. His eyebrows were shaped downward, and his brow was descending, so he really did look like a mean, angry person.

"It really bothers me that people in my courtroom are scared of me, and make snap judgments about my feelings because I look this way," he told me. "It's affecting my work. Can you help?"

In this case, I could, so I performed a face-lift. He was ecstatic afterward and his BQ shot through the roof. It was a subtle transformation—he just looked happier. He later told me that his colleagues thought he'd gotten married because he seemed so pleased all the time. They had no idea he'd had work done.

This patient was a perfect example of someone with healthy vanity. He knew what was wrong—that he looked mean due solely to anatomy—and was willing to do what it took to change it. Fortunately for most people, chances will be high that you won't need a face-lift to improve your BQ.

Everything you'll read in this book is designed to help you nurture healthy vanity and increase your self-esteem.

A Simple Tip for Nurturing Healthy Vanity

One simple step you can take in your quest to nurture healthy vanity is to be conscious of your reaction to a compliment. It should be a simple "Thank you" rather than a negative, guilt-tinged reaction, such as "This old thing? Oh, I got it on sale." If someone tells you your hair looks terrific or your dress is pretty, the effort you've put into your appearance has been noticed, and in the nicest way. Healthy vanity means you appreciate being noticed because you have a high BQ. Narcissism means you expect to be noticed because you're sure you *deserve* to be.

INSECURITY AND A LACK OF SELF-CONFIDENCE

Everybody has negative feelings about themselves—that's just human nature. However, some people are better at dealing with them than others. They're able to recognize their flaws yet continue to acknowledge their strengths so that the positives outweigh the negatives. And while they're able to admit that work might be needed, their negative feelings won't affect their daily functioning and happiness with themselves. These are the people who have a naturally high BQ.

In my line of work, of course, I see many, many deeply insecure people. Sometimes these insecurities stem from an issue that is out of their control—an extremely crooked nose, large ears, or small breasts. With the right surgery, these insecurities vanish and a formerly distraught patient is transformed overnight into a happy person.

On the other hand, I have people who come to me for consults whose insecurities stem from something much deeper. Those insecurities were caused by emotional turmoil or traumatic events, and clearly cannot be solved by a nip here or a tuck there. Deep insecurities have a much stronger hold on people's lives, interfering with their daily functioning and creating an aura of self-hatred and despair. People who suffer from this type of insecurity often become overwhelmed and feel that there are so many things wrong that they can't be fixed.

The root of all insecurity is a lack of self-confidence, for whatever reason. The first step is recognizing what your perceived insecurities are. You can do this only if you're willing to be brutally honest with yourself. Some people just need a bit of time and a piece of paper to make a list. Others might need the help of a therapist to explore painful emotional issues. Once you have identified and acknowledged these insecurities, you should be equally blunt with yourself about which of these issues you're capable of tackling on your own, and which are too complicated or difficult to manage.

For example, if you're insecure about your appearance because you need to lose a little weight, this is something you can handle on your own. However, if you lose the weight, and you're still tormented with doubts about how you look, you might want to find an appropriate counselor who can help you. This could be a social worker or religious leader at your place of worship, a support group, or a psychologist or psychiatrist.

Unrealistic Change for All the Wrong Reasons

I've found that patients who are steeped in denial about emotional pain—such as misery surrounding a bad relationship or doubts about their abilities—are often equally steeped in unrealistic expectations about what I can do for them. I've heard terrible stories of the pressure to make alterations to please others (as in, "My husband cheated on me with a younger woman, but he wouldn't have if I looked better" or, "My boyfriend likes big breasts, and he's paying for them"). All of these patients want to believe that having surgery will immediately end these problems. They want a magic bullet to transform them into someone completely different. Making major changes to yourself to address an external personal problem is not only dangerous, but also completely ineffective.

I often discuss with patients our society's ludicrous stigma against seeking counseling when you need help dealing with your feelings. If you broke your leg, you would go to a professional to get it fixed; if something is not right with your emotions, why not go to a professional to work on getting them fixed, too? Sometimes we're just not hardwired to take care of every issue in our lives, on our own. Professional therapists have studied a wide array of techniques that you can implement in your life to help you deal with psychological issues. Don't ever be ashamed to seek their help.

One of the most useful concepts that you'll learn in therapy is that you can't change other people—but you *can* work on changing how you feel about *yourself* and how you choose to act. Once you are able to incorporate this knowledge into your life—and it can be a simple or lengthy process, depending on many factors in your emotional life and family history—and are able to let go of the fact that you can't do anything about how other people behave, it can be extremely liberating and therapeutically empowering.

Changing the Negative Commentary in Your Head

Changing the recordings that run through your head is a very important element of dealing with your insecurities. They can sound like endless loops of "I'm not good enough," "I'll never get it right," "She's better than me," "I'm ugly," "I'm fat," "I'll never be thin," "I hate my butt," or "I'll never meet someone." Sound familiar?

Negative responses about yourself and the situations you are in become built in during childhood by the influential people in your life. Your automatic responses often mirror those of the people closest to you. A good friend once told me that whenever she went to visit her grandmother, she would walk into the house, say hello, and the first words out of her grandmother's mouth were, "What's wrong with your hair? It looks terrible." Not surprisingly, my friend grew up hating her hair and her appearance, and was able to overcome her insecurities about her looks only after counseling that helped her understand why her grandmother had been so negative and how powerless she had been as a child to do anything about it.

Although I often recommend counseling to those who have chronic negative commentary running through their minds, for those who deal with these negativities only in certain situations, there's plenty that you can do on your own. Here are a few tricks to make you more aware of your behavior so you can shut off the commentary and then mentally destroy it forever.

The first step in changing your negative commentary is to realize what it sounds like. One easy way to start becoming aware of these thought patterns is to listen to strangers' conversations. It's easier to judge what strangers are saying since you are unlikely to see them again and because the content of their conversations has no relevance on you or your behavior—you're merely a neutral observer. Simply listen for a few seconds to a random snippet of conversation, and based on that small sample, decide whether you think the speaker is negative or positive.

For example, if someone is trying on a new outfit that doesn't fit or is just the wrong style, a positive person will say, "Hmm, this doesn't suit me at all. Let me look for something else." A negative person will say, "Ohmigod, I look so horrible. My stomach is so flabby. I'm never going to lose any weight."

Once you start paying attention to other people's thought patterns, it's easier to become aware of your own. Compare your thoughts to those you have been observing. Do you sound like the person you were just listening to? Are your thoughts simply echoes of the negative stranger's conversation?

Become aware of your negative thought patterns, and when you realize that you're thinking this way, make a mental note of it. Then, if you need a bit of help trying to click out of a certain way of speaking, write down what you don't like so you can become more aware of it (the act of writing will make you more likely to remember this). Or, when you find yourself saying something negative, *immediately* stop and say the opposite *out loud*. You might also want to create a sort of personal self-empowering mantra, such as, "I'm a good person, or, "I'm beautiful inside and out." Say it as often as you need to. Remember, it's a healthy and good thing to think positively about yourself.

These practices will help you click yourself out of instant negative reactions and consciously respond positively. After doing this consistently, your automatic reactions will eventually shift from negative to positive, and you will begin to feel better about yourself. Your BQ will increase exponentially the more self-assured and happy you become.

Positive Reinforcement

Another very important part of building self-confidence comes from the people you have around you on a regular basis. Having someone unstintingly supportive in your life can have an amazing effect on your view of yourself. I know how incredibly lucky I am that my father was such a positive person. Without his unwavering support, I would never have gotten through college and medical school, where some of my teachers told me I was useless and stupid. During my freshman year at college, one chemistry professor actually told me that I "would never be any good, never graduate, and never, ever get into medical school."

My father's response was, "Wait a minute. You just started college— what does he know? I've known you a lot longer and I know you can do it."

Thank goodness I had such a loving and wonderful father. He made me realize that we all need to have somebody—a child, a partner, a friend, a colleague—who believes in us and who will always stick up for us . . . even when we might make stupid or thoughtless mistakes. We need to be reminded of our positive attributes during times of crisis. We need someone to call without the fear of judgment.

My father was this essential friend to me. I knew I could call him when I failed a test or messed up something else, and no reproach would come. Instead, he always made me feel better. More important, he would randomly note something I'd done well during the course of the day. That type of positive reinforcement was so effective when I was a vulnerable young man. He helped me believe in myself, which, in turn, made it possible for me to ignore hurtful criticism and take constructive criticism for what it was. To this day, when times get tough for me, I simply close my eyes and remember my father's kind and reassuring words, and this allows me to move on, endure, and succeed.

You too can feel the comfort of encouragement you received in the past. Whenever you need to, simply stop and take a minute to remember a time when you felt empowered or appreciated. If it's a particular memory, visualize yourself in that moment. Remember the scene, the smells, the feelings. If it's a general memory of someone who was always there for you, visualize that person—his appearance, the tone of her voice. Bring these comforting memories fully into your mind, and you'll be amazed at the power they have. And if ever you need more encouragement than can be provided by a memory, don't be afraid to reach out to the people in your life. There's no harm in asking for support, and the love you receive could change your life.

Believe in Yourself

One of the best things that happened to me to boost my self-confidence took place during my rotation at New York Hospital, 25 years ago, when I was a lowly medical student with a chip on my shoulder and an inferiority complex larger than the Brooklyn Bridge.

Because I was being snubbed by the other medical students who'd gone to more prestigious schools than I had, I hung out with the nurses, who were much more tolerant of my humble credentials. Plus they knew a hell of a lot more than my fellow students gave them credit for. Actually, I already knew that, as my father always advised me to listen to nurses carefully—their clinical experience can be vast since they are the medical professionals spending the most time with hospitalized patients!

Those nurses were really wonderful to me. One day, I watched as they treated someone with a bad electrical burn. The head nurse explained that if you grab an outdoor power line, the high voltage instantly travels through your body, and causes an average limb loss of 2.2 (as in two limbs that are so damaged that they'd have to be amputated).

Soon after this, the chief surgeon in the burn unit, who was a brilliant burn expert who'd written many textbooks and was viewed with awe, even by the most arrogant medical students, was leading a treatment team meeting. Basically a group of people—everyone from the chief of the department, to attending physicians, all the way down to lowly medical students—sits down together in a conference room and discusses each patient. Unfortunately for us, the surgeon's second-in-command loved torturing the residents, asking them really difficult questions to make them look stupid—just because he could.

On this infamous day, the second-in-command said, "Let's talk about the patient with the electrical burn. Here's an easy question. What's the average loss of limb for this kind of injury?"

The residents didn't know. The Cornell medical students had no clue.

"Are you telling me that nobody in this room knows the answer to this?" he went on.

By now, my friend who was the chief nurse was looking at me with her eyes on fire, so I raised my hand and quietly said, "I think it's 2.2."

The chief surgeon was so impressed that he started engaging me in more things and ended up giving me a phenomenal letter of recommendation. I had found someone who believed in me, and it completely changed my life. He, and that wonderful head nurse, gave me the self-confidence to speak up, whether I was sure of the answer or not. Having people like that on my side helped me achieve my goal of becoming the best possible surgeon I could be. I didn't want to let them down, and I didn't want to let myself down, either.

Knowing that someone believes in you will always give you an inner glow of accomplishment—and that will translate to an outer glow that automatically raises your BQ, too.

SELF-SABOTAGE AND UNREALISTIC EXPECTATIONS

Let's talk for a moment about basic emotional health and happiness, and the importance of seeing the world realistically. When you're happy and fulfilled by your life, you have a certain glow, which gives you an exceptionally high BQ. To reach this state, however, is greatly dependent on your ability to see things as they are. If you can't be honest with yourself and realistic about the important issues you face, you will sabotage any efforts to confront and deal with them—thereby sabotaging your chances at happiness.

As a plastic surgeon, I speak to patients practically every day about *their* perception of how people see them. Often, these patients treat their own external image with much more disdain than is deserved. This is especially true in New York, where the Size Zero Brigade seems to rule my neighborhood. Nearly every day, I hear women beat themselves up because they're not emaciated. Their skin is dull, their hair is thinning, their energy is lagging, and their sparkle is gone. They spend too much time fixated on their "flaws," measuring themselves against an unrealistic ideal.

Yet strangers who see them might be thinking, "Wow, that woman sure is thin. She must be amazingly disciplined, naturally skinny, or completely starving." And if it's the latter, you can rest assured that your BQ is suffering for your efforts. It is, after all, very hard to look great when you're famished all the time! Sometimes I am tempted to say to these clearly hungry people, "Please. Do yourself the biggest favor in the world, and go eat a cheeseburger!"

Comparing yourself to others and forming expectations based on these comparisons very often leads to the double whammy of not only looking less attractive—with a pinched, hard, pessimistic face and a lack of vitality—but also feeling unhappy about yourself because you can't reach the ideal you have in your mind. These negative feelings inspire pessimism and a lack of motivation that can sabotage any possibility of positive change.

These self-saboteurs who compare themselves to others soon lose the ability to see any of their positive qualities. They become focused on what they *don't* have instead of what they *do* have (and can enhance). They tend to get hung up on numbers, as in "how many years younger" they want to look, or "how many pounds of fat" they'll lose after liposuction. The problem is that there's always going to be someone younger than them, and there's always going to be someone thinner. You have to be realistic about who you are and what is right for you—not for someone else.

The point I always try to make with my patients, especially those who've brought in photographs of celebrities they wish to resemble, is that they shouldn't want to look like somebody else. They have to focus on what makes them beautiful—what distinctive features make their BQ high. Wanting to look like someone else is a terrible form of self-sabotage. It means you can't ever be happy with who you are and how you look.

A prime example of someone sabotaging herself through comparison is my patient Jane. She's 47 and has remarkably good skin for her age, as she's protected her fair skin with sunscreen over the years. She has a fairly large nose, but it's offset by large, bright blue eyes and well-defined cheekbones. She has a bit of an attitude problem.

JANE: I hate my face.

ME: Is there anything in particular that you hate?

JANE: Well, my nose is drooping. I'm getting these lines around my mouth. I have really deep crow's-feet. But mostly my nose. It reminds me of my grandfather's. By the time he died I swear his nose was down to his chin—I am not exaggerating!

ME (*after examining her*): Have you looked at your positives? For one thing, you have gorgeous skin, and your neck is in remarkably good shape, too. There's no sag at all at your jaw line. That's pretty unusual.

JANE: That's because I'm wearing five pounds of makeup. And you better take another look at my neck. The skin is all crepey. I just *hate* it.

ME: Maybe it's a little crepey as far as the lines go, but it's not sagging or drooping. You have to be realistic about what you want to do. So let's start with your nose. I could do a modest tip refinement, but it would be *very* modest because your face has a great deal of character and that's one thing you never want to mess with. You want to make minor adjustments to accentuate your positives. You have big, gorgeous, expressive eyes, so of course you're going to have some laugh lines, but that's part of your expression. A little Botox would be helpful as far as your forehead and eyebrows, but that's about it.

JANE (*not pleased to hear this*): Well, my friend Betsy is my age, and she had all this work done. Now I look really old next to her. So, really, you have to fix it.

ME: Sure, I can do these small procedures, but once you start comparing yourself to your friends, you're walking the road toward disaster. Who spent more time in the sun? Who has good genes? Who is happier and laughs more? I'm sure that Betsy has her positive and negative features, and I'm also sure even without seeing her that they're completely different from yours. Maybe she really did need a face-lift, but you don't.

JANE: But Betsy told me that all the actresses in Hollywood have face-lifts when they turn 40 and that you're supposed to do it before you're super saggy.

ME: It's true that small procedures at a younger age can often help maintain your overall look, but you can't start comparing yourself with famous faces or you're doomed. Believe me, for every example of an actress who had great work done when she was 40 and didn't really need it, I can give you ten examples of women who started too early and then couldn't stop and had too much done. And remember, photos of actresses and other celebrities in magazines are always retouched, and when they appear on the red carpet for big events, they've already spent hours having their hair and makeup done by professionals who know what will look best in photographs.

JANE (*really stewing now*): Well, if that's all you have to say, I'm going to see somebody else.

ME: I think that's a great idea. It's very healthy to get a second opinion. Most people who come here for a consultation will go see another surgeon or will be seeing me as their second or third consultation. It's very unusual for anyone to make a decision about any kind of plastic surgery or other treatments after the first appointment.

JANE: Fine. Suit yourself.

ME: But remember my suggestions, and if another surgeon tells you that you need a face-lift, I'll tell you flat out they are lying to you.

At which point Jane flounced out. No matter what procedures she'll end up having, she'll sabotage her BQ because she is unable to realistically assess her good and bad points, accept her uniqueness, and work to enhance that before going under the knife. By dwelling on what she saw as her negative qualities, she blew them out of proportion.

Being realistic about your appearance, so you can acknowledge both your positives and negatives, is one of the most important aspects of improving your BQ. This means that you need to look at yourself with an appraising eye and be honest about what you see. Doing so should help get you out of old self-sabotaging patterns of comparing yourself to others.

One of the easiest ways to figure out your strong and weak points is with a simple pro and con list. Take some time when you know you won't be disturbed, and draw a line down the middle of a blank piece of paper. On the left is your pro column. On the right is your con column. Now write. Everyone has strong points and weak points. List them all, no matter how inconsequential you think they might be.

A sample list may look like this:

Pro	Con
Nice big eyes	Crow's-feet
A good smile with white teeth	Starting to get jowls under my chin
Strong shoulders	Sagging breasts
Long fingers	Brittle nails
An okay butt	Tummy sticking out
Shapely calves	Should lose ten pounds

The key to making this list work is that there must be as many pros as there are cons. Being forced to list your good traits will stop you from focusing solely on the negative. So if there are more cons than pros, add some items to the pro column before reading on.

In comparing ourselves to other people, we inevitably set ourselves up for failure. But self-sabotage also manifests itself when we have unrealistic expectations about the amount of time and effort it takes to effect true change. People who are prone to this type of self-sabotage are easily discouraged with their efforts because the desired changes don't come fast enough. I have had many patients who have a terrible history of not following through on good programs—like diets or skin-care treatments—that could do wonders for their BQ. They give up before they have a chance to see any changes. Keep in mind that, when it comes to change, the extent of the benefits you see is directly proportional to the work you put in. There really is no "quick fix."

Be Aware of the Power of Media Messages

Ageism, which encourages unrealistic expectations, is alive and well in the mass media. How else can you explain why women's magazines use skinny little 17-year-olds to model couture gowns costing $30,000, or why these same 17-year-olds are posing in ads for wrinkle creams? And I'm not even going to get into how airbrushed those photos are. Even the tiniest imperfections are magically erased with the click of a mouse.

Because there are so few role models of a certain age, it's very hard to look at your own perfectly normal, averagely wrinkled face and healthy, toned body and not find yourself wanting. Women are bombarded with images of what a "normal" 50-year-old face looks like, when that face may have been lasered, plumped, injected—and then *still* given a heavy makeover by the airbrusher.

Believe me, I see the fallout from this Keeping Up with the Media Joneses every day in my office. Until we demand that editors stop using flagrantly unrealistic role models, I fear we'll continue to see ridiculous images that claim that beauty and sex appeal are inextricably linked with youth. Women need to realize (and be supported in their realizations) that the highest BQ comes from aging with grace rather than with a desperate struggle to turn back the clock.

GETTING YOURSELF MOTIVATED

Another important psychological component of the BQ is motivation. When my wife tells me she's too busy to work out after I've been up since 5 A.M. getting ready for the morning's surgery, seeing dozens of patients, and then running to the gym for a quick session to keep my energy high, I want to bang my head against the wall!

I'm convinced that procrastination is not a personality trait but learned behavior. If this behavior is rewarded any step of the way, it can get entrenched. And then in its own way, procrastination literally becomes the decision maker. Anyone letting inertia take over is actually making a tacit decision to *not* move forward.

So if you want to raise your BQ, you need to get motivated to act. As a start, you should make a list of general goals that you'd like to reach and why you want to reach them. List every reason you can think of for striving toward the goal you've set. Perhaps you want to be more toned, or lose some weight, or do better at work, or look less tired. Or just feel better about yourself in general. Having these goals on paper to refer back to at any time will keep the final reward in sight, thus helping you stay motivated while working.

Next, make a list of action steps that will help you achieve these goals. List the steps with specific, realistic time frames, such as three months, six months, or a year. Action steps with deadlines inspire people because they are something concrete to strive toward rather than a nebulous idea. As deadlines approach, you can check off which goals have been achieved and which have not. This can be a very rewarding process. Then you can start a new goal list.

Be proud of what you've accomplished—and *never* beat yourself up if you haven't accomplished everything in one particular time period. Simply add what didn't get done to your next goal list.

Remember the BQ is a work in progress—for life. As you get older, there will always be something to work on to raise your BQ. Instead of seeing this as a negative, embrace the possibilities and see it as a challenge. That way, you can always be encouraged and empowered by your accomplishments, and you can continue to build upon them no matter how old you are.

Here are some other hints for getting and staying motivated:

- Remember that learning any new skill is scary, so start small! For example, if you're not used to exercising, start working out in short increments, in the privacy of your home. You can put on your favorite hour-long TV show and do exercises *only* during the commercials. That will still give you about 20 minutes of exercise time. This won't be aerobic exercise, but you can certainly do a good set of crunches during one commercial, then work your arms during the next, then do lunges during the next. Gradually, your stamina and strength will increase, and you'll be able to work out for longer, and harder.

- Do the best for the level you're at. If you have unrealistic expectations about what you can do, you will no doubt fail and be discouraged from continuing your work. I ask only this: please be honest with yourself that you are trying as hard as you can. When I hear my young sons regularly say, "I'm doing my best, and that's the best I can do," it's something adults ought to remember!

- Adjust your goals as you get better at whatever it is you're doing. As I said before, start small. As your small successes add up, you can start to choose more difficult goals, and continue to raise your BQ.

- Embark on your BQ program with a friend, or even a group of friends. If you aren't alone when you decide to work on improving your BQ, you'll be much more likely to stick to the program. You can motivate each other—celebrating successes or having an understanding ear if something goes wrong. You and this group can also plan events that will motivate you. For example, you can have a swap party where you trade clothes that don't fit you or suit you, and get a whole new wardrobe.

- Reward yourself. If you reach one of your goals, you deserve to celebrate! Do something luxurious that you normally wouldn't do. Go to a spa. Get a fancy new pair of shoes. Take yourself out to a movie. Do something that is entirely for you.

- Don't punish yourself. If you're craving chocolate, eat it. But don't just eat it—savor it. Most of all, don't feel guilty about it!

Use Lists to Fine-tune Your Thoughts

I'm a big fan of lists. They help you organize your thoughts and see what needs to be done. The can also be an exceptional motivational tool—a physical representation of your goals. But it can be scary to stare at a blank piece of paper and just start writing. If this is the case for you, just write something on the page, anything to make it seem less threatening. Copy a poem. Write a thank-you note. Make a shopping list or a chore list. Just put words on paper. This will help you get going, and then the lists that are really important will start writing themselves.

Here are some of my favorite lists:

1. Counting My Blessings
2. Pro and Cons of My Own Beauty
3. Pro and Cons of What's in My Closet
4. What Makes Me Happy
5. What I'm Good At
6. What Stresses Me Out
7. What Makes Me Look Great

STRESS AND WHAT YOU CAN DO ABOUT IT

You can be wearing the most exquisite outfit, with your hair artfully styled and your makeup impeccable, but if you're stressed, you'll look it—and this will send your BQ right to the bottom of the charts. All the Botox in the world can't remove worry from your face. Also, when you're stressed, you'll always be more agitated and less patient, which detracts from your BQ.

For all of us, there are different kinds of stress: the demands of deadlines and new procedures and what interacting with co-workers can bring. Friends, family, and life in general often bring personal, emotional stress.

Just as building self-assurance through healthy vanity means taking time to care about your appearance, building emotional health through stress-busting means taking time to rid yourself of unnecessary worry. This is something I've heard endlessly from my female patients over the years—that they do not have any time to themselves to do what is needed to make themselves happier and less stressed. And when they do try to take this time, they often feel guilty and selfish. However, to take care of yourself and your stress is far from selfish—you will be more effective and successful at everything you do at home and at work. You'll be a much happier person, and those around you will appreciate that.

So, how do you manage stress?

The Boy Scout motto of "Be Prepared" is one of the most sage uses of two little words that I've ever been given!

When I first started out as a surgeon, one of the ways I helped myself manage the stress of surgery was by keeping checklists handy in the case of extremely rare complications. Fortunately, I never had to deal with these complications—but I was *prepared* for them, and in being so, I minimized my worries and was able to stay calm, cool, and collected. And when I went into the operating room relaxed, my patients invariably relaxed, too.

Now that I have decades of experience as a plastic surgeon, I don't need my emergency complications checklists anymore. I know the material inside and out. But I still prepare for each procedure by going over it in my head, every step of the way, before I start. And if the operation is to be tougher than usual, I'll sit down and read a few articles about the technique, or sometimes I'll watch a video of the actual procedure. Even the very best surgeons are never too experienced to stop learning new skills.

These mental checklists and preparations are similar to what pilots do. They go through a prescribed set of tasks prior to takeoff. They've done these tasks countless times, and know them instinctively, but they still do them to ensure that nothing has been left out. There's never going to be any room for human error in the operating room or in the cockpit.

To help you deal with your stress, write down a list of what you're most worried about before any event or what chronically causes worry in your life. Identifying your stressors is the first step in managing them. Sit down and think about your stress. If you're chronically late or find it hard to get organized, figure out what you do that makes you late or disorganized. Write it down, and acknowledge it. Then you can come up with a plan to preemptively tackle what might drive you and your loved ones into the stressed-out stratosphere.

Are your keys always misplaced? Decide to always put them in a special designated place when you get home. Do you often forget your wallet or your prescription sunglasses? Remember to pack your purse or bag the night before. Do you make a date to meet a friend and then forget about it? Be sure to write it down immediately on your calendar. Are you always the last person to board your flight because you got to the airport late? Force yourself to leave an hour earlier than you usually do!

Over time, you'll find that a small amount of preparation can prevent larger problems from forming in the first place.

Another trick in dealing with stress is plain old reasoning and the realization that you cannot control everything, which my wonderful father helped me realize. One night, before a hugely important exam while I was in medical school, I was stressed and anxious, and I told my dad how I was feeling.

He looked at me and asked, "Did you study hard?"

"Yes, as hard as I could," I replied.

"Did you prepare as best you could?" he asked.

"Yes."

"Then stop worrying. You did everything you could, and what will be will be. Now get some sleep."

His reasoning was simple and straightforward—and highly effective. Sometimes we trip ourselves into worrying about things that we have no control over, and recognition of that fact can reduce stress immeasurably.

Another great technique for managing stress is to find a hobby you love and incorporate it into your life regularly. My favorite stress buster is exercise. It took me quite a while to realize that I needed to do something intense to help manage my stress, and I started running while in medical school once I realized that it always helped clear my head before a big exam. Find a way to manage your stress by doing something you truly love to do. This will help you not only get additional pleasure from doing it but also help you *keep on* doing it.

Take my brother, a retinal eye surgeon, who is, like many surgeons, a Type A personality. He's also an avid golfer, so much so that his wife calls him a golf fanatic and I can't say I disagree with her. But he also operates on people's eyes on a daily basis to save their sight, so a high level of stress is part of his profession every time he goes to work. He once said to me that the only time his mind is completely clear of all the work-related stress is on the golf course, because of the great amount of concentration needed to play well. His competitive nature overrides his regular thought patterns, forcing him to concentrate on the game and forget about his patients for a while. It's a very healthy stress-busting maneuver.

Suggestions for Stress-Busting

It might take some time for you to find a stress buster that is effective and also is enticing enough for you to practice it. The options are endless. Here are a few suggestions:

- Do something quiet, on your own: meditate, do deep breathing exercises, take a relaxing bath, have a therapeutic massage, or listen to music

- Express yourself: sing a song, which will regulate your breathing, stop any stress-related hyperventilation, and make beautiful music; dance to your favorite tunes—alone or with a partner

- Workout: take a nice long walk or run, play a satisfying game of tennis or golf, or practice yoga

- Expand your mind: go to the movies or the theater, listen to music, read, or take a course about something you've always wanted to learn

- Take up a hobby: knit, crochet, or do other handwork; scrapbook; cook or bake; or learn to garden

- Have fun with others: play games with friends, pet a dog or cat—a proven way to lower blood pressure; play with your kids; go on a date with your significant other; and, of course, have satisfying romps in the bedroom

- Volunteer and take the focus off yourself: do community service, help out your kids' PTA, or tutor students in need

Having at least one trusted confidante to talk to, no matter when or where, is essential for stress management. This should be somebody you trust implicitly, who might not agree with you on everything but who's going to be gently honest and loving when asked for advice.

Bottling up your worries practically guarantees that the bottle will explode eventually. I used to be much less able to talk to loved ones about what was bothering me, and that was unfair to them and to me, of course. As much as my loved ones "know" me, they aren't mind readers. It took me many years to be able to open up about my needs, and I wasted a lot of time being angry over insignificant things instead of being able to let them go. Once I was better at managing my stress, I was not only a happier person (which immediately raised my BQ) but also a much better surgeon and husband.

DEFINE WHAT YOU'RE GOOD AT AND WHAT MAKES YOU HAPPY—AND THEN DO IT!

There is nothing less attractive than someone who radiates a sense of unhappiness. The BQ principle of finding your best feature and accentuating it can easily be applied to more than physical appearance. To define what makes you happy and acknowledge where your innate skills lie provide you with the information you need to choose how to spend your time and energy. Doing what makes you happy and what you're good at will raise your BQ to astounding levels.

Ben Hogan was a famous golfer in the 1940s and 1950s. In those days many professional golfers often spent more time on the "19th hole" (also known as the local bar!) than practicing. Unlike some of his colleagues, Hogan was known as a fanatic when it came to working on his game. When he started winning lots of tournaments, people remarked about how lucky he was. His response? "You know, the harder I practiced the luckier I got!"

For Hogan, practicing was more fun than playing—because it enabled him to get better at something he really enjoyed. It wasn't work, or a chore, because it helped him make a living while doing something he loved passionately. Tiger Woods has the same philosophy, as do many in other fields who excel at what they do—not just to make money but to engage themselves wholeheartedly in something they're good at and believe in.

Another example of someone with a high BQ because of the effort he expended to excel at what he liked was a successful Wall Street banker discussed in Dale Carnegie's *How to Win Friends and Influence People*. This Titan of business used to lock himself in his study for several hours each weekend to review what had happened during the previous week at work. He would recall meetings that went well and try to figure out why, and do the same thing for meetings or other projects that hadn't been successful. It's certainly an interesting habit to try to adopt, since it's basically the same as assessing your good points, as well as assessing what you don't like, and then doing something about it.

Although I know I'll never be a golfer like Ben Hogan, golf is one of my passions. When I'm having a good day on the course, believe me, everything in the whole world is more sparkling and sweet. And then on the way home I try to figure out what I did right, so I can apply the same strategies during my next round so I'll continue to improve. This not only reinforces my pleasure with my hobby, but helps improve my game and prolong the happy feelings of accomplishment.

The easiest way to pinpoint what makes you happy as well as what you're skilled at doing is to write. Make a What Makes Me Happy list and a What I'm Good At list. Write down whatever comes to mind, from the most profound to the smallest little thing. Nothing is too small to add, and everyone has many things that make them happy and that they're good at.

Your What Makes Me Happy list can include anything and everything, from the small (seeing peonies and lilacs for sale as a sure sign of spring, listening to a Bach cantata or a Kanye West song) to the large (your family, your home, a job well done).

Your What I'm Good At list can range from your work (you're a great teacher) to your hobbies (you're a great knitter, you can do crossword puzzles in ink, your banana bread is famous) to your habits (you're always on time, you're a super-safe driver, you can change your baby's diaper in three seconds flat) to your interpersonal skills (your children know they can talk to you about anything, you're a great storyteller).

I love doing lists like this—pinpointing all the good things I'm capable of—because it helps reinforce my strong points. (Of course, you can do the opposite kind of list if you want to work on some parts of your personality you're not crazy about.)

And if you want to take it one step further, you can try keeping a journal to assess what made certain projects or interactions successful or unsuccessful—just like the businessman did with his weekly review. At the end of the day, write down what happened to you and what you learned. You can do this for business and personal matters. Review it at the end of the week, and refer to it often. You'll be amazed at how much more clearly you will see your patterns of behavior—and be able to identify what's important and what isn't.

These exercises are terrific to do with your family, especially your children. They can reinforce the positives and brighten a bad day when everything seems to go wrong. They will also make you more aware of what you can do to become even better at what you enjoy doing.

It will also be a lot of fun to look back at your initial lists after you start your BQ program, as you'll certainly be able to add many new items to them. At the top should be, "I'm happy with myself." This will hugely improve your BQ score—because anyone who is happily self-confident is always going to look fantastic.

CHAPTER FIVE

Physical Health

As you know by now, a person's beauty lies in more than their physical appearance; however, you must also realize that physical health and appearance do play a part in how others perceive you. And while there's no magic bullet to improve your BQ overnight, you can certainly do many things that will help in the long run. Just remember, you can't score a high number if you don't follow the basics: regular exercise, ample sleep, good food, and daily skin care. But don't worry—improving your BQ isn't about following super-rigid rules and regulations, or kicking yourself because you were too busy to exercise for a few days, or feeling guilty because you enjoy a piece of chocolate and a glass of red wine regularly.

This chapter covers the basic physical health factors that will diminish your BQ if you don't pay attention to them. Some of these changes will be small and cost little (like getting more sleep, using sunscreen, and hydrating your skin) and will give you results fairly quickly. Others will take more time but be worth it as you'll improve every aspect of your health (eating better, not smoking, exercising regularly). Finally tackling ingrained habits you know you shouldn't have can be deeply satisfying, and will greatly improve the quality of your life.

SKIN CARE: A BASIC REGIMEN TO GET THE GLOW

According to anthropologist Desmond Morris, flawless skin is the most universally desired human feature. No single medicine or treatment can reverse complex skin problems or entirely stop the aging process, but you'll greatly diminish your BQ if you don't maintain skin health and vibrancy with a simple skin-care regimen.

Morning Regimen

1. Gently cleanse with the product of your choice. You don't need to get your face "squeaky clean"—that's actually stripping too much of your skin's natural oils. If your skin is very dry in the morning, saturate a cotton ball with a hydrating toner and use that instead. Always use lukewarm water, not hot, and rinse well. Pat dry gently.

2. Apply sunscreen. This serves a dual purpose, as it will also function as your morning moisturizer. Using both is overload, as they can clog your pores and make your skin feel greasy. Furthermore, many moisturizers advertise an SPF (sun protection factor) rating, but you need to use a lot of the cream for it to actually match the SPF number. In addition, SPF only measures protection from UVB rays (the kind that cause sunburn), not UVA—and UVA rays are what cause the damage to your skin cells, which results in premature aging and other unwanted damage.

   Without question, this sunscreen application is by far the *most* necessary step of your day, so take your time trying different sunscreens until you find one you like, with both UVA and UVB protection, and an SPF of at least 30. On sunny days, you'll need to use at least a teaspoon of sunscreen on your face, so don't skimp! (If you do, you won't be getting an accurate SPF.)

   Always apply sunscreen at least 20–30 minutes before leaving the house, as it takes that long for the ingredients to become activated. In addition, you want it to soak in before applying makeup. So I suggest you become accustomed to putting on your sunscreen first thing. Do your makeup later.

3. Apply makeup. (See Chapter 8 for details.)

Evening Regimen

1. Remove makeup. This is a must, as unremoved makeup can clog your pores, cause blackheads or pimples to form, and be extremely drying.

    Makeup removers and simple cleansers are very inexpensive, so you should be able to experiment with different brands until you find one you like. Some women like creamy cleansers they rinse off with the aid of a soft washcloth, while others prefer to use a gentle facial soap and a separate oil-based makeup remover for mascara and other eye makeup.

2. Gently cleanse with the product of your choice. At the end of a long day, it can certainly be tempting to fall into bed without cleansing your face. But not getting rid of accumulated dirt and grit of the day is one of the worst things you can do to your skin. Especially if you live in an urban area where pollution, car exhaust, and other environmental hazards end up on your skin. (Foundation and powder serve as a barrier against toxic stuff that will otherwise go straight into your pores. Frankly, it's better for your skin to be washing off makeup than washing off diesel exhaust!)

    Look for mild facial cleansers with minimal ingredients. Never use a deodorant soap on your delicate facial skin, as it can cause irritation or dryness.

3. Exfoliate with the product of your choice. This is an important step that many women skip because they don't understand why it's needed. The reason is simple: the very outer layer of your skin consists of dead skin cells. Dirt and debris will also accumulate on the surface, especially if you live in a city or spend a lot of time in traffic. If not sloughed off, this combination of dead skin cells and daily crud can clog pores and leave your complexion looking dull and sluggish.

    If you've ever gotten a pedicure, you know what I mean. You don't think twice about getting the dead skin sloughed off your feet, and you know how much softer your skin is afterward. Well, skin is skin, whether on your feet or your face! And simple, gentle washing is not enough to get rid of the dead skin cells on your face.

Exfoliation, with either a cleanser containing gentle exfoliating granules or a home microdermabrasion kit, will sweep away the crud on the topmost layer of your skin, leaving you looking a lot more vibrant. It will also help moisturizer absorb more effectively. Some women like to use buff-puff types of exfoliators, but they are usually recommended only if you have either very oily or nonsensitive skin.

Don't go overboard exfoliating. To avoid irritation, always follow the directions on your exfoliation product. It's usually recommended to use them once or twice a week at first, and then work up to every other day if needed. Also be aware of what you're using to apply your exfoliant—a washcloth with a rough texture plus an exfoliant could easily irritate your skin.

4. Moisturize. Moisturizer has a very simple function: to hydrate the top layers of your skin. So find any basic moisturizer that works for your skin type. Many good brands are at the drugstore; you certainly don't need one that costs a week's salary.

    Technically speaking, you don't need to use a separate eye cream, neck cream, and face cream, although eye creams tend to cause less potential irritation around the sensitive eye area.

Treating Blemishes

Recognize and treat blemishes as they occur, and see a dermatologist for recurring problems. Self-diagnosing skin problems via Google is not something I'd ever recommend! I can't tell you how many of my patients have gone to their computers or their facialists for advice, sometimes severely damaging their skin as a result. The worst thing you or an aesthetician can do if you have pimples or blackheads is try to squeeze them. This will not get rid of them—it will only worsen the situation and may lead to scarring.

What You Should Know about Wrinkle Creams

Anyone who's read the monthly women's magazines or gone to the cosmetics counters in a large department store knows that the companies who make OTC (over-the-counter) moisturizers and wrinkle creams, with "new" ingredients and formulations seemingly being launched every day, often make extravagant claims about their effectiveness. Some of these products also cost a small fortune.

I read the ingredient lists on these products, see their price tags, and know that much of the hype behind some of these claims defies belief, so don't fall for it! A good, basic wrinkle cream (which will have additional ingredients beyond simple hydrating moisturizers) *may* help diminish fine lines—the operative word here being *may*. Look for products with antioxidants, as they reduce the free radicals (which are highly reactive and unstable molecules that, because they damage healthy cells, contribute to the aging process, internally and externally) that can cause wrinkles. Research has shown that antioxidants can be effective in preventing fine lines from forming.

Instead of spending your money on overhyped OTC products, I encourage you to see your dermatologist and discuss whether or not a prescription retinoid (most commonly known as Retin A) might work for you. Retinoids have been studied extensively for decades and are one of the few ingredients that truly can remove fine lines and wrinkles. (It does, however increase sun sensitivity, so you must be prepared to use sunscreen religiously or your skin will fry!) None of the OTC products that contain retinol or supposedly contain Retin A can ever be as effective as a prescription-strength retinoid, as the concentration of the active ingredient must be very low for it to be classified as a nondrug, but some retinol is better than none.

Hydrating Facials

While hydrating facials can be relaxing, there is a tremendous amount of misinformation floating around in the beauty universe. Bear in mind that a facial properly performed by a licensed aesthetician can be an extremely effective way to pamper your skin. However, good basic skin care is a necessity, whereas facials are a luxury. Make sure your aesthetician has had proper training, and be wary of skin care technicians at neighborhood nail salons or day spas who dispense medical advice as freely as they do nail polish. The skin you save may be your own!

Sun Exposure: Getting Safe Sun

Okay, so blame Coco Chanel and the flappers of the 1920s for this one. Stylish women who were thrilled to throw off their stifling corsets and shed their heavy hats and annoying parasols adored Chanel's stylish jersey knits. These were no longer hothouse flowers; they were modern, energetic women! Their eagerness to flaunt their modernity marked a quantum shift from the old standard where pale skin was prized. Paleness meant they were able to afford *not* to go in the sun; they weren't out working in the fields with little to protect them save a flimsy bonnet.

Yet when women who'd always had to wear hats, gloves, and copious, floor-length garments for centuries to protect their modesty (and vulnerable skin) began exposing themselves to the sun, they got a whole lot more than a tan. They got blotches, burns, spots, wrinkles, and cancer. Sort of a huge price to pay for sitting on the beach and flaunting bronzed skin, isn't it?

Most women know, deep down, that there's no such thing as a healthy tan, yet convincing them to avoid the sun is a tough battle. There's not a huge assortment of healthy ways to get a real tan without paying the price in the form of aging, wrinkled, mottled skin.

As most wrinkles on your skin are the direct result of sun exposure over the years, using a sunscreen with a high SPF every day is, without question, the cheapest and easiest way to stop damaging your skin and raise your BQ score. And remember, sunscreen is not just for days on the beach—ultraviolet radiation from sunlight is not blocked by glass, so you can get a tan in a sunny office or while driving. Thus you need to use sunscreen every day (okay, you're excused if there's a hurricane raging outside, but that's the only possible excuse), and you need to use it properly.

When you're looking for a good daily sunscreen, choose one that protects against UVA and UVB rays. UVA radiation is what causes aging. UVB radiation is what causes burning. Bear in mind, though, that the SPF is only measured for UVB protection.

Few people know how much sunscreen to use. If you don't use the right amount and apply it as directed, you will not be getting the SPF listed on the bottle. For daily use, you should apply at least a teaspoon to your face and neck, and more for any exposed parts of your body. Don't forget your hands. For beach use, you should use up to a tablespoon for your body. Use measuring spoons to see how much this is—it's way more that you're probably used to using. Apply your sunscreen at least 20–30 minutes before you leave the house. It needs this time to activate, so if you slap it on right before running out of the house, you will basically be presenting unprotected skin to the sun. (Remember to reapply sunscreen every two to three hours if you're outside.) Protect your tender lips from the sun with lip balm containing SPF, and make sure your eyes—and the skin around them—stay young by consistently wearing fairly dark sunglasses with a UV coating.

If you just can't stand sunscreen, wear sun-protective clothing, particularly hats with wide brims. In fact, you can immediately raise your BQ if you become known for your stylish collection of hats. The Australians, who have a very high incidence of skin cancer, have become extremely proactive at encouraging use of sun-protective gear, especially for children. Too bad we're much more cavalier about sun protection in the United States.

Warning! Tanning Beds Are Dangerous

While you may like to look sunned and tan even in the winter months, you should avoid tanning beds at all costs. Tanning beds age your skin and put you at increased risk for skin cancer, particularly because they concentrate the damaging light spectrum so you'll tan faster. There is absolutely no justification for using them. In fact, a recent study published in *The Lancet*, a British medical journal, confirmed that they increase the chances of skin cancer by an astounding 75 percent!

Sunscreen is not just a valuable protection against wrinkles and freckles. Considering that skin cancer is the most common cancer in the United States, we are pretty steeped in denial about our sun worship (myself included). According to the American Cancer Society, "Most of the more than 1 million cases of non-melanoma skin cancer diagnosed yearly in the United States are considered to be sun-related."

Everyone should see a dermatologist once a year for a basic examination of moles and sun spots, as a preventative measure against skin cancer. If there is a personal or family history of skin cancer, an examination by a dermatologist should be more frequent, according to his or her recommendations.

The least invasive forms of skin cancer, squamous cell and basal cell, are curable if caught early. A simple removal of the mole or spot is usually all it takes. But even these cancers can grow and become deadly if not treated. Just the other day I was forced to surgically remove two-thirds of the right ear of an older gentleman who ignored the ulcerating lesion he'd had there for many years. It is very rare to see a squamous-cell cancer such as this advance to such a terrible state, but it was a good reminder that everyone needs to see a dermatologist immediately for any suspicious skin lesion.

The most dangerous form of skin cancer, melanoma, also has an extremely high cure rate if caught early. The bad news is that once it spreads, it is invariably fatal. Of all the reasons to die an early death, getting a tan should not be one of them!

SLEEP: MORE SLEEP CAN CHANGE YOUR LIFE

Real estate mogul Donald Trump has famously stated that he functions perfectly well on a scant three hours of sleep each night—but that doesn't mean you can, or should. Countless studies have shown that sleep is a vital body function, allowing the body to repair itself and rebuild vital connections during the night.

But I'm sure you don't need to read these studies to know what sleep deprivation does to your physical appearance. Since your skin is your body's largest organ, and since blood flow to the skin increases during sleep, surviving on a few hours of shut-eye takes an immediate toll on your BQ. Your skin will be dull and lifeless. You may have dark circles under your eyes. Your energy will be low, and there will be little pep in your step. You'll feel blah—and look it!

Ample sleep needs to be a priority in your life, not just for a high BQ but to ensure basic health, particularly as you get older. According to the American Academy of Sleep Medicine (AASM), which has an excellent Website at www.sleepeducation.com, adults need seven to eight hours of sleep every night (although many don't come close). Without it, productivity, judgment, and reaction times decline and irritability and sluggishness increase.

"The amount of sleep a person needs also increases if he or she has been deprived of sleep in previous days," the AASM adds. "Getting too little sleep creates a 'sleep debt,' which is much like being overdrawn at the bank. Eventually, your body will demand that the debt be repaid."

Unfortunately, for many the debt is repaid via the use of prescription sleeping pills. Although the occasional use of sleeping pills can be very helpful if you can't fall asleep, using them on a regular basis can lead not only to dependence on these depressants but also to dependence on a stimulant to help you wake up and have more energy during the day. This can quickly veer into full addiction and troublesome side effects that wreak havoc on your entire body and biological clock. Burnout is inevitable. A long program of either weaning yourself off these medications or more intense rehab is often needed.

Alcohol is also not an effective sleeping aid. Although it does make some people sleepy, those who rely on alcohol to fall asleep will awaken in several hours (usually four to five) later due to a rebound effect after the alcohol is metabolized and wears off. The result is more fatigue coupled with a hangover.

My favorite way to get restful, refreshing sleep is to treat yourself like a baby—by using a technique that many parents, including myself, followed with great success. They knew that what works best to get babies and toddlers to sleep is *to follow the same routine every night.*

In my home when my children were young, this meant dinner, bath, pajamas, reading a book aloud, cuddles, a little bit of talking about the day, more cuddles, and then lights out. Like clockwork, dinner was served at the same time, and everything else followed on a rigid timetable. My boys needed this schedule as much as my wife and I did! They found it soothing and comforting. We had ample proof of how effective this schedule was, as whenever we traveled out of town, disrupting their routine, they would rarely go to sleep as easily or sleep as deeply.

Although, obviously, adults have many pressures in their lives that can make a nightly sleep-time routine difficult, you can still try to create your own timetable and follow it as best you can. You can try eating a healthy snack and sipping a cup of hot chamomile tea, taking a steaming bath, reading, watching a movie (not a scary or depressing one that will keep your mind way too engaged to wind down), spending time alone with your partner, and then lights out.

When you're devising a nighttime routine, time it backward so you know how much time you'll need to do it properly. Then you'll know when to start getting ready for bed.

It might take some time to adapt to this sleep routine, but eventually it will become second nature, and you should find yourself sleeping more easily.

Here are more tips that should help you get the sleep you need:

- A hot bath is not a relaxing cliché—it really does work to calm you down and make you sleepy, much more so than showers do. If you work out in the afternoon and time is short, realize that you don't have to shower then—you can save it for later, when you can sink into some hot bubbles. Use scented bath oil (lavender is particularly relaxing) or light a few scented candles. Refuse to answer the phone or demands from your family. You need this downtime for yourself!

- Try to limit your coffee or tea consumption to early in the day, and if you do have any difficulty sleeping at night, avoid coffee or any other caffeinated drinks after midday.

- Vigorous exercise is a stimulant, and if done in the evening, it can keep you up longer. Try to work out early in the day, or at least before dinner.

- Try to avoid heavy dinners, especially if they're very rich or spicy. These may keep you up because your body is digesting the food and blood flow to your stomach prevents deep sleep from occurring.

- Create a calming sleep environment with a white noise machine, heavy window curtains, or even a fan, to help blot out street noises or other distractions. Use soft cotton sheets, thick comforters, and lots of pillows to turn your bed itself into a cozy and inviting haven.

- Use your bedroom only for bedroom activities, which include lovemaking and sleeping. Just as it's not a good idea to have a television in your children's bedrooms, it's not a good idea to have one easily accessible from your bed. It's too easy to turn it on and get distracted. If you do have one in the bedroom, try to place in it a cabinet with doors that shut, so you can shut it out!

- If you prefer to read before sleep, have your lamp easily accessible. The last thing you want to do as you're dropping off is have to get up to turn off the light!

EXERCISE: YOU'VE GOT TO MOVE IT

If you want to own your beauty, you need to own your body as well. Which means that if you want to have a high BQ, you've got to move it—you must exercise. Although it can be very tempting to lounge in front of the TV every night, especially after a long, hard day at work or in the house, the great paradox of exercise is that the more you do, the more energy you will have. It will also help you sleep more deeply, which in turn will help you look better.

Getting in shape and staying in shape takes work—not a huge amount, mind you, but enough to get your blood flowing so muscles get toned and your skin glows. A fantastic side benefit to exercise is weight loss, but you shouldn't be moving it simply as a means to manage your weight. You should be moving it as a basic, necessary component for good health. Few women with super-high BQs get those scores (and keep them) without the discipline and commitment to incorporate regular exercise into their lifestyle. The exercises in Appendix D will help you in your quest to get and stay fit.

Firm and strong bodies are sexy, and a nice figure can complement a beautiful face. But firm and strong bodies don't come naturally to most of us (certainly not to me!), despite what you might read about super-thin models and actresses in women's magazines. It is entirely possible to be both skinny and unhealthy, too.

Finding the Right Movement for You

The bottom line for your BQ is that you need to find some physical activity that you really like and that suits your body's strengths. For example, if you tend to have joint problems, running is not going to be recommended but swimming or biking likely will be. If you enjoy your exercise, you'll be much more likely to stick to it because it won't seem as much like work. You don't have to go to a gym if it's either too expensive or doesn't suit your personality. A lot of my patients have told me that they don't like the competitiveness that's often found in gyms, or just don't like to work out around a lot of other people, particularly if they're new to exercising.

And then there's the time factor. Getting to a gym, changing your clothes, working out, showering and changing, and getting home can be extremely time-consuming. If that's the case, you can easily exercise at home (which is where the exercises in Appendix D will also be helpful). There are countless exercise DVDs available, and you can learn how to belly dance or samba, do yoga, Pilates, or weight training, in the privacy of your living room. Even better, you can exercise at whatever time of day suits your schedule, or even work out with your kids—a win-win for the entire family). Try renting different exercise DVDs or a Wii (along with the Wii Fit or one of Wii's other fitness programs) until you find a program that's enticing enough to do regularly.

Why I Like the Gym

I always exercise in a gym, and my trainer, Jill Livoti, explains why going to one is beneficial if the time and cost factors are realistic for you:

- Focus. It gets you out of the house and clears your mind. You'll be able to ignore the phone, computer, TV, and other distractions.

- Inspiration. You can get inspired by other people of all ages and shapes working out.

- Teamwork. If you decide to play on a team that meets in a gym, you can use the facilities, shape up without thinking about it, and have the satisfaction of exercising with a group of people. Plus you won't want to let the team down, so you'll be much less likely to miss your regular workouts.

- Proper technique. You will learn how to perform the exercises properly to maximize results and prevent any injuries.

- Safety. If you're injured, there will be immediate support and help.

Another ridiculously easy exercise option is walking, an activity anyone can do during the day. It costs nothing, and has no downside (unless your shoes don't fit properly). You can do it year-round, with your family members or friends, and you should be able to find an indoor area, like a nearby mall, for walking if the weather makes it difficult.

Don't forget about something you'll likely have nearby: the stairs! During the course of the day, whenever possible, take the stairs up and down as many floors as possible. This burns a surprising number of calories and tones the large muscle groups of your legs and buttocks. You can also do isometric exercises and stretching while sitting at your desk, and stand up to stretch every hour or so.

Other good cardio choices are bicycling, boxing (especially great for toning arm jiggle and tightening butts!), dancing, jumping rope, power walking, running, skating (or Rollerblading), skiing, or swimming.

I also recommend sports like golf or tennis, which might not be as aerobically challenging as running or swimming, but are satisfying since you're playing with partners. I don't cancel my golf dates unless I'm treating someone with a medical emergency. It's not just to avoid letting my partners down—I also need to clear my head, walk around in the fresh air, enjoy my friends' company, and get rid of pent-up stress by the very satisfying act of swinging a club and hitting some little white balls! It's an even more satisfying day if I avoid the golf carts and walk, as traversing an 18-hole course will add up to several miles. If possible, try to carry your clubs in a lightweight bag rather than driving around in a golf cart, as this will strengthen your arms, shoulders, and legs, and burn even more calories.

Whatever form of exercise you choose, have it be one that you truly enjoy. If you start working out a certain way and either get bored or fed up, you'll be much more likely to find excuses. Mixing and matching different activities is an ideal way to work all the parts of your body, stop yourself from clicking into autopilot (where you won't be working out efficiently or productively—ever see the people in the gym, riding the recumbent bikes while reading magazines? They might as well not bother!), and most of all, never get bored.

Don't Compare Yourself to Anyone Else

However you exercise, don't compare your body or your progress to anyone else's. When you're changing your body, you're on a journey, and the progress you make and the route you take to get to the desired goal is yours alone. You're not going to get a body like Madonna's unless you spend 30 years working out for as many hours a day as she does.

Genetics also plays a role as those with a specific body type, called mesomorphs, will always put on muscle faster and easier than others. Your body will always have one tough zone that is tougher than others to shape up—for some women it's their buttocks, for others their bellies. And once you start to exercise and lose weight, you'll usually notice it first in your face, then in your upper and lower extremities, your calves, your forearms, and only then in the places where you really want to see results!

Getting in the Routine

One tip for anyone starting to exercise is to hire a certified personal trainer for a few sessions to teach you correct form, which is crucial, particularly for exercises with hand weights or that work your abdominals. If you're on a tight budget, you can split the cost with several friends. Having a good trainer show you the correct moves will speed the pace of your program, ensure you reap the maximum benefits from whatever you're doing, and help prevent any injuries that could result from doing the exercises incorrectly.

Another very important part of starting an exercise program is prioritization. Only you can decide how to organize your life so that exercise becomes a habit as ingrained in your day as brushing your teeth and taking care of your skin. I find that getting up an hour earlier and getting my workout done makes me feel great and have more energy, which helps me tackle whatever tasks lie ahead. Plus, I don't have to dread working out after a long day at the office.

The most important thing when figuring out what time to exercise is that it has to work with your schedule. I have a friend who exercises regularly, even though her job necessitates numerous long airplane trips. When she travels, exercising is not always an option, so she's created her own system, where she'll work out for 15–30 minutes longer for several days before and after her trips, and it all evens out in the long run.

If owning your beauty is now a priority, you'll find the time. It's time you need to spend on you. And once you start exercising, the fact that you're taking the time and making the effort will immediately raise your BQ, even if you're only adding a few minutes of exercise to ease yourself into a program. The dividends are not just an improvement in physical strength and stamina but in every other aspect of your life, too.

Move It to the Music

Music gets me moving during my workouts. I've put together a music file on my MP3 player, with my favorite up-tempo songs that stimulate the senses and allow the time to fly by. It's easy enough to compile your own workout playlist with songs that you love—and that you know will get you moving. You'll find, as I have, that you'll easily fall into a higher exercise level as you move to the beat and rhythm of the music, improving both your workout and your mood.

NUTRITION AND YOUR RELATIONSHIP WITH FOOD

My uncle Phil met my aunt Ida walking down 116th Street in Manhattan one hot summer's day when he was 16 and she was 14. It was a great love story—they met so young and then were married and nearly inseparable for 60 years. I never got tired of my uncle telling me about his first memory of my aunt, seeing her on her way to church, wearing a beautiful summer dress with a large bow low on her back. As she walked by, he couldn't help notice that bow bobbing up and down in rhythm with her steps. He just could not stop thinking about that bow! Of course, it took me a while to realize he actually was referring to her beautiful derriere, but in a very sweet way.

When it was time for my uncle to retire, he and my aunt moved to Florida. At one point she went away to visit relatives for a few days, so my uncle was left to his own devices. Since he was a terrific cook, he made himself dinner every night. Even though he was on his own for this short period, he set the table with the good silver, the good china, a heavy crystal wineglass, and a linen tablecloth and napkin.

One of those nights, just as my uncle was about to sit down to eat, a neighbor came by to check on him. This neighbor gaped at the beautiful table setting and made a snide comment that if the table hadn't been set for only one, he might have thought my uncle had been about to seduce someone!

My uncle was not pleased to hear this. "So what if I'm eating alone?" he told his neighbor. "Why shouldn't I enjoy myself? Eating is a pleasure." And that was the end of that.

I love that story, because it says so much not just about my beloved uncle but also about how important it is to respect and enjoy how and what you eat.

Developing a healthy relationship with food is very important for raising BQ. A woman who eats well and within nutritional guidelines for her age and her body will always be more attractive. While delving into the intricacies of eating a nutritional diet are beyond the scope of this book, there are a few essential points that will guide you toward a healthier relationship with food. If this relationship is currently tumultuous, I suggest that you consult a registered dietician, who can not only help you understand the emotional aspects of eating but also counsel you on an eating plan based on science. Fad diets won't help you with these aspects of nutrition and will most likely fail in the long run. If you simply want to learn a bit more on your own about nutrition, there is a great deal of helpful information at reputable Websites like www.nutrition.gov or http://fnic.nal.usda.gov.

How We Think of Food

As my uncle knew, when you sit down at a properly set table, and when you eat slowly and savor what you're eating, you engage in what's called mindful eating. You aren't obsessing about food. In fact, the more slowly you eat, the less likely you are to overeat—both because you will be emotionally satisfied with your savored cuisine and because you'll be allowing your body enough time to feel the effects of what you have already eaten.

I find that mindful eating is also inspired by exercise. People who exercise become far more conscious of their bodies and what they're putting into them for fuel. If you're spending all the time and energy to have your body run at maximum efficiency, eating a less-than-optimal diet isn't going to work anymore.

Just remember that what you put into your body is reflected in your outer appearance. If you don't eat enough, your skin will be dry and lifeless, and your body will be bony and haggard. If you eat too much, you'll be putting yourself at tremendous risk for serious medical conditions, such as diabetes, and even a shortened life span.

The process of eating is as important as the food itself—if not more so. This is a belief that was instilled in me early in my childhood. I have indelible memories of waking up early on Sunday mornings to the smell of my mother slow-cooking pasta sauce and meatballs and sausages. Sunday dinner was a tradition in our home; however, eating the gargantuan meal was merely a ruse for our entire family of uncles, aunts, cousins, and friends to come together and catch up.

Those cherished Sunday dinners strengthened the bonds of our family. Since my mother passed away, I have tried to instill the traditions of cooking as a family with my two boys, and during the holidays my sons and I manage to make our own scrumptious lasagna from my mother's recipe (and nearly wreck the kitchen at the same time). The kids love the process: making the sauce, assembling the noodles, and of course nibbling as we cook. Their look of pride and satisfaction when we serve the lasagna to the family is priceless.

My uncle Rocky used to say to me as a little boy, "Bobby, I truly feel sorry for those people who were not born Italian. Look what they're missing!" Try to create your own family eating traditions, which are as much about togetherness, love, and commitment as they are about food. Nurturing through a shared meal cannot be underestimated.

So think about how and what you eat. Mindlessly picking at food from a takeout or microwave container while watching TV is not a good way to nourish yourself. Prepare your meals with love. When you eat, think about the flavors, the textures, the aromas. Be thankful for the food you have and delight in eating it. Only with an appreciation for all aspects of food can you develop a healthy relationship with it.

SMOKING: BUTT OUT

When I first met a very smart, sassy, and adorable woman named Valerie, I was struck by the proverbial thunderbolt and fell head over heels in love. I knew that she was the woman that I wanted to spend the rest of my life with. Except for one little problem. She smoked!

Early in our relationship, I told her that as much as I was crazy about her, I just could not live with a smoker. I went down the list of health reasons, and then admitted that kissing an ashtray was not for me. Valerie listened carefully, then she stopped, for me, on her own. I was never so proud and flattered. Now I *had* to marry her!

It was the best decision I ever made, and putting out her cigarettes was one of the best decisions for her health (and her BQ) that Valerie ever made, too. Because here's the warm smoke and cold hard facts: Smoking is one of the worst things you can ever do to your skin and body. The American Cancer Society warns that smoking is responsible for nearly one out of five deaths in the United States, as well as at least 30 percent of all deaths from cancer. It's also a major cause of heart disease, aneurysms, bronchitis, emphysema, and stroke. It worsens pneumonia, flu, asthma, and is linked to other conditions like peptic ulcers, gum disease, cataracts, and osteoporosis. It can damage a woman's reproductive health and have dire consequences for babies.

Smoking decreases the blood flow, which means you'll get a lesser flow of vital nutrients to your skin when you need them most. Unquestionably, it does the same thing to your heart and lungs, along with causing cancer. I get so frustrated when my patients spend large sums of money, time, energy, and recuperation on major procedures to look fabulous, and then go out and instantly start undoing everything they've paid for when they light up.

According to the American Cancer Society, most smokers want to quit, but only 5 percent actually succeed. I wish there were a surefire method to help all smokers quit for good. Many of my patients have tried hypnosis, acupuncture, and nicotine gum and patches, to varying degrees of success. There are also FDA-approved drugs, Chantix and Zyban, that can be effective. They do not contain nicotine but work by blocking the nicotine receptors to the brain. Studies show success rates as high as 44 percent, so they're definitely an option you should discuss with your physician. It should go without saying that, as with all prescription medications, these drugs may have serious side effects, so you need to be informed about all possibilities.

CHAPTER SIX

Personal Presentation

Charisma—it's an intangible, magnetic force that simply makes you want to be near someone. That someone might be tall or short, loud or quiet, gorgeous or homely, sensitive or aggressive. Their clothes may be bargain basement and their makeup negligible, but what they all have is that something that effortlessly seems to flow from them. Movie stars possess it. So do politicians and models. So do stay-at-home moms in Topeka, Kansas, and beach-going moms in Miami. It's a certain way of walking, or gesturing, or wearing clothes—of creating a compelling presence.

It's nearly impossible to put your finger on the precise quality that gives these people panache. You know it's there, but you can't explain it. And while some of this intangible quality comes naturally, there is much—charm, poise, affability, and some pleasing personality traits—that can be studied and learned. Applying the techniques in this chapter, as well as in the rest of the book, will help enhance your charisma and give you that je ne sais quoi.

MAKING A GREAT FIRST IMPRESSION

There are two well-known sayings about first impressions: "You never get a second chance to make a first impression" and "First impressions matter." And you know what? Both of these are true. Your first impression sets up the relationship you will have with the person you're meeting. And while it is possible to change people's feelings about you, it's easier to start out on a good foot. Plus, being able to easily meet someone with confidence increases your BQ more than you can imagine.

First impressions are not just about how you look but also about how you treat people and how you present yourself. That includes your initial greeting, the expression on your face (hopefully a smile!), your handshake, the scent of your cologne, your posture, and making eye contact.

On their own, these are very small things, but when put together, you have less than a second and only one chance to make a sensational first impression. Which means, fortunately, that tiny little tweaks to your personal presentation can reap you huge rewards. Your personal presentation is an outer reflection of your inner state of mind, so you should always strive to reconcile the two and always try to look your very best.

Making Eye Contact

I deal with first impressions practically every day at my office. And after more than 20 years, I can tell you that my perception of a new patient begins with eye contact. A woman not comfortable in her own skin will not look at me directly.

Eye contact is key to how people see you. It shows confidence, trust, and self-esteem, or a lack thereof. If you're walking down a crowded city street, meet a stranger's eye, and flash him a confident smile, you will instantly be perceived as a happy, self-assured person with a high BQ. Confidence—especially if you're confident because you know you've worked extra-hard to look sensational—is a wonderful thing to see. Knowing how and when to make eye contact, acknowledging another person, responding in a pleasant way, and using body language to your advantage is a trait that everyone with a high BQ has mastered.

So how do you develop this skill? It's simply practice. Try to make eye contact with the people who are closest to you. Then expand your practice by making eye contact with those you know, then those whom you aren't as close to.

A Good Handshake

My father was an old-school internist, the long-lost kind of doctor who thought nothing of making house calls in the middle of the night. His patients just loved him. He always had a knack for knowing exactly how to touch these patients. He had a very gentle way of taking a pulse or a temperature, always seemed to know who needed a hug, and spent time with them when they needed it. He listened. He always had a kind word.

As sick as many of his patients were, they always felt better after a visit with Dr. Paul Tornambe. His touch told them that he cared, that he was there for them, and that their pain and worries were acknowledged. He once told me that he would always take a patient's pulse for two reasons: the first was the obvious reason; the second was to reinforce the strong doctor–patient bond. The touch of a skilled physician can mean so much more than a hastily written prescription and a quick dismissal.

Touch can convey so many things, and since handshakes are usually your first form of physical contact with any new acquaintance, they are very important. If someone's handshake strikes you as weak and limp, or too hard, or too intimate, this first impression will likely stay with you. So take care to shake hands firmly. Look the person in the eye and smile at the same time. Say your name with confidence, and use the other person's name in the ensuing conversation. Remembering and using a person's name while you talk is an excellent way to begin building a relationship with someone you've just met.

Posture, Posture, Posture

One fine day I was walking down the street and saw, from a distance, what I thought was an absolutely gorgeous woman. She had a beautiful coat on, topped with a stylish hat. She was carrying an expensive handbag, and talking animatedly on her cell phone. But as I drew closer, I could see that her lovely features were contorted in pain, and then I realized that she was walking very, very slowly. I looked at her feet, and immediately figured out why.

Her glorious designer shoes were torturing her. Not only was she slumped over but she was walking in tiny mincing steps as if she'd just stepped out of the Imperial Court in China, her bound feet unable to carry her weight. Talk about a fashion victim—those shoes were *killer*, all right! They killed her feet, they killed her posture, and they killed her BQ.

As soon as I passed this woman, I immediately thought of one of my son's pediatricians, a wonderful doctor in her late fifties. Where the other physicians in her practice dress down, she dresses *up*. I always marvel at her, dressed in those gorgeous outfits that always seem unruffled even after she'd spent a very long day dealing with sick kids and their stressed-out parents. And she always wears heels. I find that astonishing, as I could never wear anything but the most padded, comfortable shoes in my office!

Naturally, this doctor has an exceptionally high BQ. So, after one visit, my wife couldn't contain herself and said to her, "I don't know how you do it."

She looked at my very tall wife, shrugged, smiled, and said, "Well, darling, I don't have your height. What do you expect me to do?"

The most potent weapon we have in our arsenal when it comes to presenting ourselves is how we sit and stand. Posture is everything. You could be dressed perfectly, with fabulous hair, great makeup, great *everything* . . . but if you're going to walk with a slouch or an ungainly stride (or ridiculously uncomfortable shoes), you'll ruin the whole package.

There's just something incredibly important in carriage. Any woman with a great way of moving will appear youthful and lithe. If she's got small breasts, walking tall will make them appear larger. And she'll look ten pounds thinner when she stands up rapier straight. She'll *always* raise her BQ score then.

If you want to test this out, go to a busy street at lunchtime or to the mall on a crowded weekend, grab a seat, and watch people walk. It can be fascinating! You'll see for yourself how attractive women can ruin or raise their BQ by the way they move, whether they shuffle or strut, keep their heads down or look straight ahead, keep their shoulders rounded or slumped, or squared back with an aura of competence and confidence. Any woman who slumps and slouches will instantly age herself.

You don't need to be a trained dancer to be able to walk with strength and grace. When I was a child, my female classmates often walked around the room with books balanced on their heads. The boys would snicker and laugh, but those girls knew what they were doing. Their spines were aligned. Their core muscles—the ones that give you a flat stomach—were engaged. And they got into the lifelong habit of walking straight and tall.

It's not difficult to learn how to walk, but it is actually difficult to learn how to walk *well*.

You'll want to do posture checks throughout the day.

Standing: Whenever you're standing, particularly if you're waiting for someone or something (such as a train or an elevator), be conscious of your posture. It's all-too-easy to slump, hunch over, or let your abdominal muscles go slack. Good, strong posture not only makes you seem taller, but also helps you work your muscles more efficiently.

1. At home, stand sideways in front of a full-length mirror. This will help you become aware of how you naturally stand.

2. Tighten your abdominal muscles. This will automatically engage your core, which is the site of the most strength in your body.

3. Square your shoulders. They shouldn't be pulled back unnaturally, but should feel comfortable yet with a little tension in them.

4. Keeping your chin up isn't just a figure of speech. With your chin up, you can't help but look straight ahead when you're walking, automatically improving your posture. (Keeping your chin up is also a great idea when you know that someone is taking your photograph. It will make your neck look longer and camouflage any sags or lines. If your chin is down, your nose will look longer and far more droopy than it really is.)

Sitting: If you work at a desk or in front of a computer, you'll need to consciously remind yourself all day long to check your posture. It is terribly easy to slump, especially when you're concentrating at work, and this can wreak havoc on your back (and the rest of your body). Set the alarm on your computer to beep every hour to remind you to check your posture.

1. Get an ergonomic chair that is properly adjusted for your height relative to your desk and/or computer.

2. If you can't get an ergonomic chair, get a hard pillow, and place it at the small of your back. This will remind you to sit up straight.

3. Use a footrest if you're short. Wiggle your feet and circle your ankles as often as possible.

4. As often as you can remember to—but at least once an hour—take a deep breath and pull your abdominal muscles in. Sit up as straight as you can and lift both your arms straight up, over your head. Stay that way and gently feel the stretch for a moment or two.

5. Stand up and stretch, too, at least once an hour.

Here are more tips to keep in mind when you're working on your posture:

- Like my elementary school classmates, try walking with a thick, square book on your head. Look at your posture when it's balanced comfortably. *That's* how you should be standing! You can do the same thing when you're sitting at your desk.

- Wear shoes that fit and that are well-made. (Cheaper shoes tend to have little or no arch support or breathability.) If you have to walk any distance, try to wear shoes that don't start hurting the minute you put them on. If you're crazy about high heels, only wear them to special events and for the shortest time possible.

- Exercises that work your core and strengthen your back are essential to good posture. See the abdominal and back exercises in Appendix D.

- While standing, you don't need to carry the weight of the world on your shoulders—in the form of your handbag. Surely you can toss out some of the heavy things in there. It's practically impossible to walk straight and true when the shoulders are imbalanced.

- Yoga or other exercises that teach you how to breathe properly are a terrific way to improve your posture. A good instructor will make sure you are properly aligned when you're in the class, so you'll know how it feels to be standing or sitting correctly. Try to work on standing poses that involve balancing. Then as your muscles get stronger and your breathing techniques improve, you'll find it much easier to stand straight without having to think about it.

- If you find yourself still slouching, ask one or two people who see you often to notice your posture and remind you if you're slipping. It can take time to correct your posture, especially if you're trying to undo a lifetime of slumping!

The Importance of Personal Scent

How you smell is as important as how you look—if not more so, as scent will always provoke a visceral reaction. Smelling a delicious whiff of vanilla and cinnamon can trigger memories of the first time you made cookies with your grandmother. Inhaling the fresh, clean scent of fir trees can make you think of being with your cousins on Christmas Eve. Coconut oil can transport you back to the beach where you had your honeymoon, and baby powder can take you right back to the first time your child smiled at you.

Just as with a handshake, if you meet someone whose scent strikes you as "off," you will likely never forget that initial, visceral impression, even if you get to know that person and end up really liking him or her. The first step in smelling good—which probably doesn't need to be said—is basic cleanliness. Showers and baths are the most important thing you can do for your personal scent. From there, you can add perfume, lotion, or deodorant to enhance your smell.

If you want to wear perfume, make sure to sample a lot and find one that smells good, isn't overpowering, and suits you. Smelling great and feeling good about your personal scent will make you happy and raise your BQ yet again.

To find the perfect perfume, there are a few essentials to learn. The first is that perfumes are made from three notes: top (what you smell immediately), middle (what it quickly develops into), and base (the longest lasting). After application, it usually takes at least 30 minutes before you smell the base notes, which may be completely different from your initial impression. So you should never buy a perfume on first whiff, as you'll only catch the top note. Try a perfume several times before buying it, and keep sniffing it for at least an hour after you've applied it. Good perfume salespeople know that this is necessary and should encourage you to test and then come back later. They also understand that choosing the right perfume takes time.

Next, remember that everyone's body chemistry is unique, so perfume doesn't smell the same on everyone. It's great to ask someone what she's wearing if you really like it, but be aware that it might smell completely different on you. Also, some women, like my wife, don't "hold" scent very well, which means it quickly wears off. Valerie found that wearing men's fragrance takes care of that problem. Many women do prefer the more unisex fragrances that have a citrus or woody base, and are not sweet or floral. They're rarely as heavy or powerful (or as expensive) as women's fragrances, so it's easy to experiment with different ones.

If you only want a little bit of fragrance, use scented body lotion, cream, or deodorant. And don't forget your hair. Great-smelling hair is a subtle and lovely touch to your entire package, especially in intimate moments.

And finally remember that perfume is one of those items that you often get what you pay for. Cheap perfume won't last, and it's made from synthetic ingredients that can alter their properties after it's applied to your skin, so it can end up smelling obviously fake. Good perfumes may be expensive, but they do last for a very long time.

After you've chosen the perfect scent for you, the application should be simple. Just dab or spray the perfume on your pulse points— the wrists, neck, inside the elbows, and behind the knees. These points are the warmest spots in your body, and because perfumes are made with oils, they react well to warmth, releasing more scent.

Never apply perfume to your hair since the oils in it can mix with the oils in the perfume and change the scent entirely. Also, avoid spraying perfume on your clothing, as it will most likely stain.

And remember, your scent should never walk into the room before you do. Less is more. If you can, alternate scents. If you use one for too long, your nose may desensitize to it, and you might put on way more than is needed.

BEYOND THE FIRST IMPRESSION

Once you've learned the art of making a good first impression, you need to maintain the new relationships you've just forged. Besides the obvious—being a caring and loyal friend or a trustworthy acquaintance—there are a two major aspects of keeping a relationship interesting and desirable: speaking and listening. Mastering these two skills will help keep you in everyone's good graces and make you a welcome member of any group.

Speaking Well

A very important part of your BQ is how you speak. A powerful speaker can hold a huge crowd in his or her hand—and oddly, what's said isn't nearly as important as *how* it's said. Watch an old newsreel of World War II speeches, and you'll notice right away how political dictators often twist the skill of speaking to their advantage. So do actors, which is why going to the theater or to see a good movie can be such an exhilarating experience. They know that a person who might not strike you as attractive on first impression can magically be transformed into the most delicious, seductive person alive, speaking to you as if you were the only person in the room, solely through the power of voice.

There will always be people who have a unique quality to their voice and hone it to their advantage. Jacqueline Kennedy Onassis was well known for this. She had an unusually soft voice, one that didn't quite match her physical persona, which was smart, sleek, and sophisticated. It always made a huge impression on those who heard her.

Keep in mind that how you hear yourself and how others hear you will always be different, because the sounds made by your voice are formed in your voice box, which is internally connected with your ears. This internal connection relays sound through your head, which enhances or downplays certain elements of it. The voice you hear is a combination of the sounds that come out of your mouth and the sounds that travel internally from your voice box to your ears. This is why people who speak very loudly or very softly often don't realize it, because to them it sounds normal. One of my very best friends has an incredibly booming voice, and the volume increases whenever he's telling a story that he's excited or passionate about. I often feel like nudging him when we're at social gatherings, because he truly doesn't realize that he's unwittingly coming across as strident.

While I know about the interplay of the voice box and ears, I am still surprised to hear my own voice. I often dictate patient notes into a recording device, and when I listen to the tapes, I think, "That can't possibly be me! I don't really sound like *that*, do I?" It can be downright shocking to hear yourself, especially if you're not in the best of moods (such as, perhaps, after yelling at the kids for spilling bright red punch all over the white sofa, or after barely escaping an auto accident, or while frustrated with colleagues at work).

A friend of mine reminded me about how important tone of voice is when she reported that, when she asked him to do something innocuous, her five-year-old said to her, "Mommy, why are you using your angry voice?" She thought she was being perfectly neutral, but her son didn't perceive it as such. His bewildered comment made a very strong impression on her, and she was working hard to turn it down a notch when talking to her little boy—and everyone else who might get the wrong impression about her, thinking that she was a little bit too strident when she'd thought otherwise.

Along with the natural timbre of your voice, which is something you're born with, everyone has certain quirks of speech, whether it's their accent, the way they emphasize certain words, how quickly or deliberately they speak, their enunciation, or the fluidity of their sentences. These are learned, not genetic, behaviors. And everyone has traits they might not be aware of, such as adding "you know" or "like" to nearly every sentence—which can be annoying and instantly lower their BQ.

Learning how to modulate your voice can take a bit of deliberate effort. The first thing you have to do is be aware of what your specific quirks are, so you can start to listen for them. (Recording yourself is the easiest way to do this.) Ask trusted friends to be blunt with you about what they like and don't like in your speech patterns.

If you're not happy with the sound of your voice or how you speak, don't be too hard on yourself, as making changes to something you normally don't think about won't happen overnight. If it turns out that you find it too tricky to change your speaking patterns, a vocal coach might be able to help. Or try singing lessons. They'll teach you how to breathe properly (and they're fun, too, because everyone can learn how to sing). Even yoga will help you learn how to breathe deeply, which is the easiest way to change how you use your voice.

Another easy way to raise your BQ is to have a laugh in your voice. It's not only a very youthful trait, but sounding happy and full of fun automatically makes listeners smile. (Many good comedians, while telling a joke, will chuckle just prior to the punch line, which is a very effective technique, especially if they're looking for more laughs.) They'll feel great listening to you—which means your BQ will go way up in their estimation.

Being a Good Conversationalist

While crafting a pleasant speaking voice is a great first step in your quest to become a desired acquaintance, knowing how to listen well and ask questions are the keys to being a great conversationalist. You can be the most interesting person in the room by simply inspiring others to talk. This will immediately raise your BQ—and the BQ of the person you're talking to.

The basics of being a good listener are all about making the person you're talking to feel special. You are face-to-face, so the power of your expression is amazing. Make sure your face portrays what is going on in the conversation. Be conscious of your expression, so you aren't inadvertently scowling during a happy story or smiling during a serious one. Also remember to hold eye contact with the other person in your conversation. Wandering eyes indicate that you are bored or uninterested in the conversation. This can really kill a relationship, as it comes off in our culture as exceptionally rude.

Body language and posture are other important parts of being a good conversationalist. How you stand, sit, or hold yourself can make people feel comfortable and secure. Try to remain physically open to the person you're talking to. Don't cross your arms across your chest, turn away, slouch, or fidget. Also try to remain about an arm's length away. Being too close to the person you're talking to can make discussions extremely uncomfortable.

Another habit that's extremely common and very rude is interrupting. My wife and I have had many conversations about this, as she chronically interrupts. Valerie has very sweetly tried to explain that sometimes her thoughts are just tumbling out faster than she means them to. And while this can be more acceptable with your loved ones or close friends, the habit of interrupting can quickly turn people off from a conversation with you.

Aside from body language and listening skills, the most important aspect of being a good conversationalist is knowing how to ask questions. This is one of the key points in the deservedly famous Dale Carnegie book *How to Win Friends and Influence People.* Nearly everyone loves to talk about things that interest them, and if you can ferret out what their true passions are, chances are extremely high that this person will become animated and loquacious.

At a dinner party not long ago I put the Dale Carnegie practice of asking questions into action. I was seated next to an actor of some renown, who'd started his career as a rapper. I asked him how he changed gears in his career so successfully and he proceeded to tell me the very interesting story of his career and his life. I enjoyed listening to him, nodding and occasionally chuckling as he continued talking throughout dinner. I found out later that he thanked our dinner host for seating him next to such an interesting conversationalist—meaning me! People love to talk about themselves or their family, and your stock will go up with them by just showing a simple interest in what they have to say.

Asking questions accomplishes two very important things. First, it shows the person you're talking to that you're actually paying attention and are interested in what they're saying. Second, it gives you the opportunity to turn a boring conversation into a more exciting one. In a dull conversation, instead of merely nodding politely, ask specific questions. Press for more details. See what you can learn. Then try to steer the conversation toward something that might interest you, too. You can even turn boring conversations into a game or personal challenge by seeing how long it might take to turn the bore you're stuck with into an interesting conversationalist by asking the right questions.

Learning how to ask questions is easy. Watch how journalists on television ask provocative questions and press for interesting answers to liven up an interview. Observe people in your life who you would consider good conversationalists. Also, prepare ahead of time with, perhaps, five interesting yet general questions, which may be altered to fit the particular subject to liven the conversation. Afterward, if your questions didn't do the trick, figure out what you might ask at the next social situation. You never know what might ensue!

Here's something else to think about: When you are deeply engrossed in a conversation, everyone else in the room is going to be looking at you and wondering exactly what you're talking about. Not only will you make the person to whom you're listening feel important and the center of your attention (which is always a positive thing), but you've immediately transformed yourself into an extremely interesting person—and raised your BQ—merely by being polite!

STYLE BASICS—CLOTHING

One of the reasons I developed the BQ program was after seeing so many lovely women in my office who did themselves a huge disservice by downplaying their innate good looks, thinking themselves "old" (and acting it) and not understanding some basic style principles that would weed out the unflattering clothes in their closets and remove years from their appearance. Of course it doesn't hurt that I'm married to a former model, Valerie Mazzonelli, who's shared her insider knowledge about fashion, style, and beauty since I've known her, making a certain style consciousness a regular part of our household.

Valerie was discovered by John Casablancas of Elite Model Management in the bargain basement of Alexander's department store when she was 16. She modeled for Elite in Europe for seven years, and it was there that she learned to appreciate and emulate different kinds of beauty. European women seemed born with a sense of chic and had the self-confidence to carry it off.

Another perk was working with world-class fashion editors and stylists during photo shoots, who showed her what suited her best; listening to the best makeup artists, who taught her their many tricks, step by step, so she learned to replicate the looks with a deft hand; as well as strutting down the catwalk during fashion shows, where she learned how to carry herself and have presence, even if she was having an off day. Faking it can work!

After moving back to New York, Valerie signed with The Ford Agency and worked through her pregnancies. But her seemingly effortless style isn't a matter of luck—it's due to her hard work. Once she figured out what best suits her figure, she was able to develop a wardrobe of clothes and accessories that maximize her strengths and minimize her flaws (yes, even models have cellulite). Fine-tuning these basics means she knows she'll always look great, whether she's taking the kids to school or going with me to a formal event.

Though she is married to me, she's never had any plastic surgery—or any desire for it!—and has a super-high BQ. You'll have one too, as her advice infuses the following sections.

The Whole Package

Coco Chanel allegedly once said, "Dress badly; notice the dress. Dress well; notice the woman." She was certainly onto something. All women with high BQ scores know that looking your best isn't about wearing a fabulous outfit or having a spectacular piece of jewelry. It's always going to be about the whole package—how you dress, how you walk, how you smile, and how you choose to show yourself to the world. The key to a high BQ is to know your positive and negative traits and work with them to create your unique beauty.

The only way to identify your positive and negative features is to stand in front of a mirror and take a good hard look. Be blunt. Assess your face, hair, and figure. Then write down what you like the most and what you like the least. Perhaps you have large hips, but you've got slim ankles. Or you might be busty, but you've got a small waist. You might have long fingers or a shapely neck. Everyone has at least one spectacular quality, and that's what you should highlight. For an example of a pro and con list, see Valerie's list below.

The next step is to figure out what you can do to accentuate each of the positives and work with each of the negatives. This woman can avoid wearing incredibly tight-fitting skirts or pants that will accentuate her belly and derriere, and perhaps forgo sleeveless shirts. But that doesn't mean she can't wear nice skirts with belts that will help define her hourglass shape, with shirts or sweaters that draw attention to her beautiful breasts and décolleté. When she focuses on her great skin and hair, too, anyone who notices her will be paying much more attention to her top rather than her bottom.

Valerie's Positive/Negative List

Positive Qualities

- I'm healthy
- I have great skin
- My hair is still pretty incredible
- I have long legs, nice shoulders and arms, a good neck and décolletage, and I'm tall and slim

---

Valerie's Positive/Negative List

Negative Qualities

- My big feet
- Cellulite on my butt and upper thighs
- Weaker abdominals after two babies
- Awful fingernails

What I Do about It

- Being disciplined about skin care, with no exceptions! Always wearing light and fresh makeup when I leave the house.

- Going to a wonderful hairstylist and colorist, to tame the roots that are all-too-obvious without treatment. Using a good shampoo, conditioner, and the right styling products for my hair's texture helps, too.

- Accepting that I will never have nice, dainty feet; finding fabulous shoes to help disguise their shape; regular pedicures.

- Keeping up my exercise routine while lying to myself that it will actually get rid of the cellulite dimples (I know it can't, but hey, I'm trying!); consoling myself with the fact that most women, even supermodels, have cellulite.

- Diet and exercise, and strengthening exercises for my abdominals.

- Regular manicures, in nail salons or doing it myself, and occasionally sleeping with hand cream and gloves for cuticle care. (Luckily, my husband finds that sexy!)

- Dressing appropriately for my body type to hide all the above flaws. For instance, I'll wear bikinis if at my ideal body weight, and wear slimming one-piece suits if not.

- I'll also accentuate the positives, wearing high heels to accentuate my long legs, on special occasions, or a nice-fitting top to show off my toned upper body.

Doing a blunt assessment might sound simple, but it's not always easy to take an objective look at yourself, especially if you've been trying to lose weight. It's often easier to harp on the negatives than to think of yourself as a work in progress. This can be especially difficult for women who, after having children, find that their bodies never quite get back to the way they were pre-pregnancy.

Developing your BQ and keeping a high score is a lifelong process. Only after you've accepted yourself the way you are *right now* can you figure out what you might need to do—to change it or enhance it to have the highest possible BQ.

It can actually be quite liberating to say, "You know what, these ten pounds aren't going anywhere in the near future. So what? I'll make them look good on me. And if I'm going to be a size 14, I'm going to be the most stylishly put-together size 14 I can possibly be."

Developing Your Style BQ

Many of my patients spend a lot of time sighing with regret that they don't have supermodel looks or a size zero figure. They're often looking for a radical and painful solution to a problem that doesn't really exist—or exist at the level they think it might. What I always tell them is that they might not be models in a magazine, but they certainly have the tools to look their best and to style themselves in the best way possible. They're fully capable of creating a high BQ and developing their own trends.

Knowing what items of clothing best suit you will make getting dressed and ready to go an easy process. Plus it will save you thousands of dollars since you won't be buying clothes you'll never wear again. So how do you get to the point where you can instantly assess what clothes will suit you best?

One of the best ways is by getting professional help. A neutral and knowledgeable third party is an invaluable resource, and nearly every large department store in America has a free on-site personal shopper. All you have to do is make an appointment, be honest about your height/weight and what sizes usually fit, and discuss your needs and your budget. Once you put on just the right outfit, you'll have that Eureka! moment, and you'll instantly be able to build the rest of your wardrobe and look around it.

Fit Is Key

I have an acquaintance who is extremely overweight, yet he hides his size well because he wears the most impeccably tailored suits I have ever seen. His size becomes almost irrelevant. So although I fear for this man's health, I have to say that his BQ is as high as it gets. He knows what works for him, and boy, does he work it!

Here's where you can take a lesson from the men in your life. They know that a superior quality, superbly tailored, and constructed suit will last them for decades. Certain items are worth a heftier price tag, as you'll get far more value for your dollars over time.

The better the fabric, the longer it will last. This is true for upholstery, and it's true for clothing. Don't spend a lot on casual wear—spend the most you can afford on signature pieces that will become the foundation of your wardrobe. A suit with trousers and a skirt can have infinite variations once you start to style it with accessories and blouses. But if it isn't well made, it will quickly start to fall apart once you take it to the dry cleaners.

One of the reasons women avoid getting good-fitting clothes is because they want to wait until they're at their ideal weight before giving their wardrobe an overhaul or spending the money on good tailoring. Yet wearing clothing that's too small will produce that "sausage effect," accentuating lumps and bumps and lowering your BQ. This not only emphasizes the negatives and brings down your confidence, but it can also affect your motivation to lose the weight, making the problem seem more overwhelming than it is.

Bottom line: Don't put off buying clothes for when you lose weight. And definitely don't buy clothes for the someday-they'll-fit scenario. If you need those pants right now, buy them. Make sure they fit perfectly on the body you have today. You can always go to the tailor as you lose weight. Or buy yourself another pair of pants.

Don't forget that monthly weight fluctuations are inevitable, so most women have a wardrobe comprised of different sizes. Try to keep the range of sizes to a minimum, because if you don't, you're giving yourself an excuse not to lose weight (if that's your issue). Being confident, and accepting your body as it is now, will keep your BQ high.

Another reason that so many women dress in ill-fitting clothes is because they look at the labels instead of at the garment itself. Forget about labels. Especially the *number* on the labels. I know it might be hard to believe, especially in our teeny-weenie-size-obsessed fashion

111

world, but size truly is irrelevant—because there is absolutely no industry standard about sizes anymore. Valerie is five-foot-nine and quite slim, yet her clothes run from size small to the occasional large. It's very frustrating, but this annoyance proves that how clothes *fit* is far more important than what size is printed on the tag.

Once you've gotten past the size issue—and believe me, if the labels bother you, it's simple enough to cut them out—then what you need to concentrate on is fit. Clothing that fits you properly will *always* look good. It's as basic as that.

Men who wear suits knows this well. They think nothing of having an off-the-rack suit tailored, and that's a service any good men's store automatically provides. Women are much more unlikely to expect the same kind of attention. Which is a bit crazy, because this means you might overlook buying something that is right for you and your budget, simply because the pants might be too long or a little too snug in the back.

Clothes that are nearly perfect but a little too large should easily be fixed by a competent tailor. Clothes that are a little too snug, however, usually can't be fixed, unless there is a lot of fabric in the seams or waistline that can be let out. You shouldn't buy shoes that don't fit well, no matter how glamorous. And never buy something that doesn't fit merely because it's on sale! In fact, you shouldn't buy an outfit that doesn't fit right unless you are absolutely certain that tailoring will provide the proper adjustments.

Proportion

While proportion may sound like a simple concept, it's actually quite tricky. But the importance of understanding proportion cannot be overstated, as it is the essence of knowing what will work best on your specific body.

Proportion is something I've studied during my entire career as a plastic surgeon, because so much of what I do has proportion at its heart. When patients come in with photographs of noses or lips or eyes that they like, it's up to me to explain how the proportion of their own facial structure and features might mean that Julia Roberts's wide lips or Michelle Pfeiffer's pert, thin nose would look totally wrong (and decidedly fake) on them.

People often associate being proportional with a body type, but being tall doesn't mean that your body is any more proportional than that of a shorter person—it just means that there's more of you. Bodies come in all sizes and shapes, and all are equally likely to be disproportionate. Ideally, having a body with good proportions means legs are longer than the torso and a torso that fits the frame.

So while it might be great to have nice long legs, you might have a short torso, which will make it hard to find a pair of jeans that flatter your shape. Jeans are all about the rise (the length between the waistband and the top of the inner thigh or crotch). If anyone who is short-waisted wears a pair of low-rise jeans, the waist band is likely to hit them in just the wrong place on the hips, leading to belly bulge and making the hips and buttocks look inadvertently larger or disproportionate to the waistline.

Tops are generally easier, as long as they are not strongly contoured or tightly fitted. But if, for instance, you have fantastic broad shoulders but a squarish shape without a defined waist, jackets will likely be hard to find as they are usually contoured at the waist.

As you're always going to be looking to accentuate your positives, once you figure out what your proportions are—and this is where someone with a trained eye, such as a personal shopper or a tailor, will be a huge help—you'll know what to do to highlight the good and disguise the less good. Good style will help make you proportional or help you embrace and highlight the disproportions that are attractive and distinctive—such as really long legs or huge, pretty eyes. Knowing and being comfortable with your body will make your BQ instantly rise.

Here are a few of the common disproportions people complain about and hints about how to use style to your advantage:

- Let's say you have a long, thin torso but short or thick legs. This can easily be rectified when you wear any shoe or boot with a heel (not too high!). Wearing boots with a stacked heel will give the illusion of length, too.

- If you're short-waisted, you need to be aware of where the waistline of your clothing sits on your body. Best bets are tops that end below the waistline, hitting the top of the upper hip bone. This will instantly elongate the line.

- If you are fortunate enough to have an hourglass figure but not a swanlike neck, you can wear a form-fitting top, turtlenecks, or a stylish scarf.

113

- If you're all legs, it may be difficult to pull off a dress with a defined waist, but you can enhance your proportions with dresses or tops that have an empire waist, or with a great shift.

- If you're very busty yet slim in the hips, you're lucky because you can wear tighter skirts or pants coupled with a loose-fitting or shiftlike top, unless you want to highlight your cleavage. (If not, a supportive minimizing bra will be one of your wardrobe staples.)

As for designer clothes, instead of concentrating on someone else's definition of a classic, you can create your own by wearing clothes that always give the illusion of balanced proportions coupled with impeccable fit. Don't be a slave to fashion—be a slave to your BQ!

Wardrobe Basics

When Valerie modeled in Europe, she spent many hours people watching. Often, what she saw was no more complicated than a basic uniform of a tailored or softly silken shirt; jeans or trousers that fit perfectly; a crisp coat or jacket that hit at the precise right part of the hips to give the illusion of slimness; an artfully arranged scarf; flat shoes or boots with a small heel; hair that didn't appear too "done"; small stud earrings and perhaps a gold or silver necklace; a swipe of black mascara; and a little bit of neutral lipstick.

Endless variations on this uniform worked for women of all ages, because the basic principle was clean lines, harmoniously accented by accessories that complemented each other but were unobtrusively sexy and smart.

So let's take a look at basics that will enhance your BQ, too.

Suits: A well-constructed suit, with a jacket, skirt, and trousers, is the basis for any woman's wardrobe, even if you don't work at a job that necessitates business attire. The color is a matter of what you like best, although simple neutrals will get the most mileage and be the most fun to accessorize. A good option is to have at least two suits if you can, one light and one dark, with different weights of fabric for those who live in seasonal climates.

One of the best things about a suit is its versatility, as it can be mixed and matched with all other items in your closet. The options are endless, as a good suit will travel with you, attend services at your house of worship, go to meetings, and then out for the evening. Wearing a smartly tailored suit jacket with jeans is instant casual chic, as is wearing tailored suit pants with a gorgeous sweater. Add a silky or lingerie-like top and you have an instant sexy dinner date.

Trousers: Think of Katharine Hepburn's sexiness as she strode across a Hollywood sound stage in one of her beautifully tailored, high-waisted, wide-legged pairs of pants. Pants that fit can make a short woman look tall, and a tall woman even taller. Pants that don't fit, however, will make your butt look big, your hips look vast, and give you a pain in the belly.

It is a rare woman indeed who can buy a pair of trousers off the rack and have them fit perfectly. Of all the items of clothing you'll own, trousers are the most difficult to fit—so be prepared to have them tailored or altered for a perfect fit. This will make even an inexpensive pair of pants look custom made. But if your trousers are so ill fitting that tailoring starts to cost more than the garments themselves, you're better off with a different pair.

Jeans: Valerie is convinced, as am I, that many women love jeans because they're simply part of the culture of American fashion. Everyone seems to wear them, right?

But jeans are all about fit—and not everyone can wear them, as denim is the kind of durable fabric that doesn't have any give to it. For the best fit, look for jeans that have at least 5 percent spandex in them, as this bit of stretch can make all the difference between pain and perfection.

As with everything, the fit is key in jeans. If you have a flat butt, wearing jeans that pump you up and add some shapeliness to that area can work wonders. If your butt and/or thighs are on the large side, you'll want to look for a cut of jeans that is less form fitting through the derriere and has a lot of give. If you carry your weight in your belly, try on a lot of different pairs that may ride higher or lower in the hips—you won't know which is best for you until you try them all on. One of the most important hints I can give you is to pay close attention to the placement of the pockets in the back. Good placement can make all the difference.

Just remember that how jeans fit is extremely idiosyncratic, and you should plan on trying on a lot of different pairs. If you can't find a pair that makes you look good, don't buy them!

115

Dresses: Is there anything more wonderful than a dress that accents your curves in all the right places? Think of Marilyn Monroe in that iconic shot, standing atop a subway grate with her voluminous white skirt blowing every which way. Actually, Marilyn had a lot of negatives to her figure—she was small but big-boned, busty, and gained weight easily, particularly in her belly area. But that white dress accentuated all her positives. Her bust was firmly supported by a halter style; her waist was nipped in; and her derriere was round but firm, encased in an opaque panty attached to the dress.

I think it's a shame that so many women choose separates when there are so many options to highlight their positives in a beautiful dress. Dresses can be far more comfortable and forgiving than pants and skirts.

You should have a few casual dresses, as well as a more formal one, for each season. A little black dress is a classic, and will always be appropriate (except, perhaps, to a summer wedding!), and can easily be dressed up or down with a fantastic piece of jewelry (whether it's a pricey string of pearls or a brooch you picked up at a flea market for $2.50).

Skirts: As with dresses, there are countless choices of skirts available, but it takes a good eye to make them work. Don't expect the skirt of your suit to fit you perfectly off the rack. A little bit of tailoring can do wonders, and make skirts much more comfortable to wear. Skirts are particularly recommended if one of your best assets is your legs.

The best skirt length depends on your age, body type, and style of the skirt. If you are 65 and still have the gorgeous legs of a 30-year-old, unfortunately a mid-thigh miniskirt is still extremely age-inappropriate and an excellent way to instantly lower your BQ. For most women, the most flattering length is just above the knee or at mid-knee.

Shirts, Blouses, and Sweaters: Basic blouses are a wardrobe essential. A basic blouse has a classic, tailored cut to it. It can be in whatever palette is complementary to you and your outfit. The quintessential basic blouse is a crisp button-down white shirt. Pairing this with a black pair of pants or jeans for casual time will flatter everyone. If you have a great neck and shoulders, don't cover them up with turtlenecks—look for V-neck or off-the-shoulder styles. If you're busty, blouses with darts and shaped seams will help minimize. If your upper arms could be firmer, long sleeves or three-quarter-length sleeves will make this a nonissue.

The thicker the sweater the more weight it adds to your body, but that doesn't mean women who have large breasts or hips should avoid them. It just means you should look for sweaters that have the right length for your body. Many sweaters are cut on the short side, so they hit right at that unflattering spot on most women's hips. Keep trying them on until you find one that hits either above or below the widest part of your hips.

Undergarments: An essential part of helping your clothes look great is to buy undergarments that fit. If your underwear doesn't work, then whatever you put on top of it isn't going to work either, no matter how gorgeous the outfit or how trendy the style.

Most women are wearing the wrong-size bra, which not only won't look good but also can be painful and annoying, especially if there are underwires digging into your skin after a long day. Almost all department stores have a fitter in the lingerie department, so don't be shy about asking for help.

You also need to be aware of the dreaded VPL—Visible Panty Line. A VPL can ruin even the most spectacular outfit, yet it's hard for most people who don't have three-way mirrors in their homes to assess precisely how they look from the back, and how their clothes move as they walk. Find a way to check this—either by yourself or by asking someone in your home.

Many of my patients are fans of Spanx, the modern equivalent of the girdle—except they're incredibly comfortable. And they really do work. They smooth your hips and buttocks, and they also help with your posture. I actually recommend Spanx to my patients after liposuction, as they are comfortable and still provide the support that is required to help swelling dissipate after the operation. Still, Spanx should not be considered an everyday item.

Incorporating Color into Your Wardrobe

It always amazes me when so many of my patients come into the office wearing black. Sure, a little black dress is indispensable, but many of these patients seem to be afraid of color. How do I know? I wear a bright blue tie (blue being my best color), and they compliment me on it, saying, "Oh, I could never pull off a color like that." Sure they could . . . if they tried!

A woman with an adventurous sense of color will generally have a high BQ—because wearing bold colors is a hallmark of women with confidence and a sure knowledge about which hues best suit their complexion, hair color, and mood.

Using Accessories to Improve Your BQ

It once would have been unthinkable for a stylish woman to leave the house without hat and gloves. And while it's not such a bad thing to be freed from the tyranny of style dictates that insist you *must* be seen with certain accessories, I do miss seeing the hats and gloves and coordinated handbags of my mother's generation. They're very *I Love Lucy* (and how I loved that show!).

A woman with a high BQ knows how to add just the right accessories to her outfit. This could mean a hat, gloves, scarf, boots, tote bag, handbag, and umbrella on a damp and chilly winter's day. Or it could mean nothing more than an heirloom gold brooch pinned strategically to simple dress.

I've seen plenty of women with stunningly high BQs even though they must wear ugly uniforms at work. They'll be wearing a great ring or pair of earrings, a nice watch, and comfortable yet good-looking shoes or boots. Their hair and makeup and nails will be perfectly groomed. Their posture will be impeccable. They might have to wear clothes to work that don't match their personal preferences, but they'll still *own* the look, because they know how to style the whole package with the precise use of accessories.

The only rule to accessorizing is to have everything coordinate. This doesn't mean the various pieces need to match (which can often be overkill), but they can't fight each other. This can distract from the whole package. So if you have a look-at-me handbag, don't diminish its impact with a flamboyant shawl or loud necklace.

Jewelry: Archaeologists will be the first to tell you that the women of ancient times went to their graves adorned in their finery. But because jewelry can have so much dazzle, you've got to be judicious in how you wear it. Flaunting your wealth with Elizabeth Taylor–sized diamonds is guaranteed to lower your BQ score, because that's all about ego, not beauty.

The key to wearing jewelry is to not let it wear you. If you're planning to leave the house with a spectacular piece, keep your clothing, makeup, and hair very simple to showcase it.

Or perhaps you might want to buy a signature piece to call attention to one of your great attributes. If you have beautiful long fingers, get some great rings that will showcase their allure. If you have a lovely neck, add a necklace. If you have strong cheekbones, a pair of diamond ear studs will direct the eye toward their sparkle. Plus, looking at an amazing piece of jewelry that makes you happy is a good way to improve your mood.

You don't have to spend a fortune on jewelry as there's an incredible world of costume jewelry available. Have fun finding pieces that coordinate with your outfits—and become an essential element of your own signature style.

Shoes: On *Sex and the City,* Carrie Bradshaw woke up one day and realized she'd spent enough on shoes in her lifetime to have made a down payment on an apartment. Shoes are an endless source of fascination for many women. As with clothing, if the shoe doesn't fit, don't wear it. It's impossible to have a high BQ if your feet are covered in blisters, or if your shoes are so ludicrously high that you can barely walk. This doesn't give you license to wear sneakers with business attire, a BQ-lowering trend in the 1980s. There are plenty of comfortable yet stylish shoes.

That said, Valerie insists that sometimes—and only sometimes!—attaining beauty does involve a bit of discomfort. Wearing those drop-dead gorgeous shoes can be as unpleasant as plucking your eyebrows or doing a number of crunches, but if the event is special enough (and the shoes killer enough), swallow the pain while knowing that you look extra-fabulous—but only for a short amount of time.

Handbags: Handbags have become the accessory du jour, and that's reflected in the wide array of choices (as well as some ridiculous prices). If you do a judicious bit of shopping, you can find great bags in a huge range of styles, colors, and prices, from thrift shops to couture to Target.

While a top-quality handbag will last for decades, some of them have gotten so big that they can overpower your look (and leave you lopsided), particularly if you're petite. If you do need to carry a lot of stuff, consider using a smaller purse for your valuables and a stylish tote bag for larger items. Valerie has raided her mother's closets for vintage handbags that have remained stylish over the years.

Sunglasses: Jacqueline Kennedy Onassis did more for sunglasses than anyone I know. She loved oversized glasses with dark lenses. As she had a strong, square-shaped face, they fit her perfectly, and became part of her look (and her mystique).

Use a wardrobe of different sunglasses to raise your BQ, as they'll instantly change your look. They're one of the least expensive and easiest ways to accessorize. They also protect your eyes and skin from the sun, so there's no downside.

Hats and Gloves: I love seeing women who know how to pull off wearing a hat. Their confidence always raises their BQ. Just be prepared for the attention because hats can be tricky. They need to not only fit your head but also add the right kind of proportion to your look. If your hat is truly incredible, as with jewelry, keep the rest of your outfit simple.

Gloves are also an item that some people are still crazy about, and as they're no longer a must-wear item, particularly in the summer, wearing gloves to accent an outfit is a trademark of confident women with high BQs.

Dressing for Your Age and Size

Part of making a good presentation to the world and feeling good about yourself is styling yourself in an age-appropriate way. Remember that trying to look youthful—rather than the best for your age—will always make you look older. That doesn't mean you're consigned to the Dowdy Department and have to throw away your favorite pair of jeans once you hit 60. It just means that if you're 60 you don't dress as if you're still 25.

How my patients dress is one of the first clues I notice about their self-image. An older patient who dresses like her granddaughter is likely to have a hard time being realistic about her surgical options or results. Whereas a woman who has accepted that her miniskirt days are long gone, and who understands her limitations as well as her strengths—particularly her resilience—is one who gets her pleasure in life from things more important than articles of clothing.

Instead of raiding your teenagers' closets, try flipping your age to your advantage and discover an entirely new way to approach your style. You can still have fun shopping and styling yourself to keep your BQ high whether you're 17, 47, or 77.

As for understanding the BQ of your size, I look to the British cooking show host and author Nigella Lawson. She's known for having a sensual attitude toward food, and it shows. She's got an hourglass figure with ample cleavage—and she wears clothing to flatter these assets. Her daytime look is often a snug sweater, a wide belt, and a slim skirt. Her nighttime look features dresses that emphasize her gorgeous décolleté, particularly with cinched waists. She's a perfect example of a woman whose BQ would go way down if she *lost* weight!

Clearing Out the Closet

You only need to have clothes that fit you *now*. Not the clothes that fit you ten years ago, and not the clothes you want to fit into.

Clearing your closet from all the clothes that don't fit can be a hugely cathartic experience, but it's not one that a lot of people can do easily. I'm not talking about getting rid of anything that might have sentimental value, like the jeans you were wearing the night you met the man you ended up marrying, or your mom's favorite party dress. Or anything so stylish that it's a perennial classic.

Don't clean out your closet until you're sure what your new look is going to be. Then take everything out and start sorting. Get rid of functional clothes that you haven't worn in more than two or three years, or anything that's never fit well, or that you're holding onto only because it was expensive.

If you're having trouble doing this, ask a trusted friend to help you. In large cities, there are professional decluttering people who will help you, for a fee.

Once you've forced yourself to get ruthless, it can be very satisfying to donate the clothes, especially if they're barely worn. Local charities will be grateful for them. So will friends. Valerie knows lots of ladies who have "swap parties" all the time, which is an excellent way to get rid of something that's a really nice article of clothing but that just doesn't work for you. Exchanging it for something that fits you better is an ideal situation.

In America, performers Jennifer Hudson and Queen Latifah are equally radiant examples of knowing how to dress to flatter their beautiful full figures. They're proof that women who aren't super-skinny can be drop-dead gorgeous. They keep their BQ high once they figure out how to accentuate their positives to deflect the eye away from the negatives.

Valerie once went to a bridal shower of a large-sized relative. One gift after another was opened, with practical, not-sexy items for the trousseau. Valerie had bought a beautiful lace nightgown and matching robe. When the bride-to-be opened Valerie's gift, she lit up like a Christmas tree. Everybody in that room was so happy, even though they'd been afraid themselves to acknowledge that this woman was a sexual person just because she was big. How ridiculous was that! Here was a woman comfortable in her own skin, about to marry a man who loved her exactly the way she was, and why shouldn't she celebrate her sexiness? She *owned* it.

No matter what your size, you need to own it. Not own the body you might have had when you were younger and several sizes smaller, but the body you have *right now*. Only by taking responsibility for your body can you assess it properly, find clothes that fit it properly right now (as opposed to fitting the body you used to have or might want to have), and stop shying away from camouflaging it in clothing that signals that you've given up trying to look good.

The most common mistake larger ladies make with clothing is to wear things that are oversized, or that skim the body instead of hugging it. But caftans, big shirts, and oversized dresses actually add the illusion of *more* weight. Well-fitting clothes will always make you look slimmer, as long as you're wearing the right undergarments to keep your lines smooth and sleek.

STYLE BASICS—HAIR

Your hair is like a halo, framing your face, and from a distance, it's the first thing someone will notice about you. As a result, if you want your BQ to remain high, you need to be honest about your hair and your relationship to it. To help, New York hairstylist and colorist Michael Valenti contributed to this section.

The Emotional Aspect of Hair

The relationship you have with your hair is inextricably intertwined with your self-image. It is part of who you are. Whether you let it grow, cut it, style it differently all the time, dye it, or let it remain the same for years, your hair is an ever-present part of you—an outward expression of your inner idea of yourself.

Because your hair makes a statement about you, the decision to cut or dye your hair can be extremely emotional. In fact, I'd say that it's comparable to a face-lift—with the only (and large) difference being that hair grows back reasonably quickly, and a face-lift cannot be undone. A haircut that suits you perfectly can raise your BQ in a way that few other processes can quickly do. In fact, a good, stylish new haircut can be as rewarding as a good face-lift!

Obviously, if you find it impossible to change your hair over time, you need to ask yourself what you're holding on to. If you're 52 years old and still wearing your hair the same way you did as a teenager, there may be an underlying issue that needs to be addressed. And that's not an easy thing to do—but once you do it, it can feel as satisfying as clearing the closet clutter and taking the steps necessary to move on.

Cutting your hair or changing its color is an act of bravery. It can be immensely freeing if you like the results—or devastating if you don't. Fortunately, color can be redone and haircuts will always grow out!

Hair Styling Basics

The best way to find a good hairstylist is through word of mouth, but only from someone whose hair is similar to yours and styled in a way you like. You can make a friend or stranger happy with a compliment on her hair, and get a good recommendation at the same time!

Be realistic. Sure, every woman wants a glorious mane, no matter what color or texture she's born with, but taking pictures of haircuts you like that would be impossible to do with your hair is guaranteed to make your hairstylist wary of your opinions. A good haircut takes face shape, body shape, hair texture, and your needs into consideration.

An honest consultation with your stylist is enormously important, especially if you're thinking of changing your look. Be upfront about how much time you have to style your hair in the morning, as well as about your budget and how often you can afford to visit the salon. Take into consideration whether or not you are handy with your own hair, because when you're home you'll be styling it yourself.

Never let a stylist (or friend!) talk you into anything. It's always better to make small, incremental changes than go for something drastic, which might take years to grow out.

Be very careful with any process or treatment that uses strong chemicals, such as perms, as they can damage hair and scalp. Do your homework before deciding to go for any major hair processing treatment, as it's a commitment—of time, money, energy, and potentially problematic results. You need to make sure that your stylist is highly experienced and highly recommended.

There are many excellent options, such as Japanese hair straightening, with results that last for months. A friend of Valerie's had this done, and prior to the procedure was unhappy about the many hours involved and the exorbitant cost. Afterward, however, she was transformed. Her hair had been extremely thick and wavy, and she could barely style it with a blow dryer. Now, her hair was straight and glossy, like a shimmering waterfall. Her BQ went through the roof. Not only was she ecstatic about all the time she saved on her hair every day, but she knew that she would walk out of that house with her hair looking great. To her, it was an extremely wise investment—in time and happiness.

Most women look great if they go a little bit shorter as they get older. But that doesn't mean you need super-short hair; in fact, the shorter and more intricate the cut, the more you need to maintain it and need regular trims.

A universally flattering length is usually somewhere between ear length and shoulder length. This gives you the versatility to style your hair easily. Having hair all one length can be limiting, and for most women, a good haircut will have some layers cut into it to give hair movement and softness. It's this movement that will give you the most youthful appearance.

Don't overwash your hair. It's time-consuming, drying, and hell on your hair color. Use the least amount of shampoo that does the job effectively, and only a tiny bit of conditioner (too much will leave your hair lank).

If you're going through a major change in your life, be wary of changing your hair drastically. I've talked to many patients who went through breakups and divorces, and the first thing they did was cut their hair. They wanted a completely new look, as if they were singing "I'm Gonna Wash That Man Right Outa My Hair" like Nellie Forbush in *South Pacific*. You may want to make small, subtle changes, such as highlights, at first. Think of this time in your life as weeding a garden instead of pulling up all the roses.

About Hair Color

I see a lot of patients—men and women—who have truly terrible hair color in a failed attempt to look younger by covering their gray.

They know that deciding to color their hair means high maintenance, but they haven't found the right attractive and youthful shade, so their hair pulls their BQ score way down.

Hormonal changes mean that, for the overwhelming majority of men and women, hair loses its color as it ages. It can also change texture and become thinner. Hair color not only restores color and luster, but also coats the hair shaft so hair appears thicker. These are two wonderful aspects of coloring your hair, but you must realize that it's a major commitment.

You don't have to make a drastic change to your entire head of hair once you start to go gray. It's easy enough to be subtle, with perhaps a few highlights blended in, which, if you're Caucasian, can be done easily as hair is never just one color. So, for example, if you have very dark hair but fair skin, you might want to think about chestnut tones. Medium brunettes can try for warm golden tones. Blondes can add highlights. Be aware that red on gray is the most difficult color combo to maintain; it often needs to be pumped-up with a color-enhancing shampoo between visits. Don't forget to consult your colorist about the best products for your hair and hair color before spending your money!

I know that many women are afraid that once they start coloring their hair, they won't be able to stop. While it's true that coloring your hair might mean time and energy and money, it can also be a lot of fun—as well as something that will make you look sensational. The power of color can change your entire look—instantly. When the color is fabulous, your entire head is going to look fabulous, too, even if you're having a blah, colorless day.

For me, seeing women who've changed their hair color always takes me back to the scene in the movie *Moonstruck,* when the character Loretta, played by Cher, decided to color her hair to remove the gray before a big night out at the opera. The transformation was striking, as this attractive but matronly bookkeeper morphed into a more vivacious and beautiful woman who nearly bowled over her beau, played by Nicolas Cage, when he sees her transformation. It doesn't have to happen only in the movies!

Proudly Gray: Some of the women with the highest BQs I've ever seen have absolutely radiant gray, silver, or white hair—as Meryl Streep famously did in the film *The Devil Wears Prada*—and the confidence and skin tones to pull it off. But maintaining gray, silver, or white hair still takes a lot of time and patience.

And not everyone goes *fabulously* gray. How good you'll look depends on hair texture. Sometimes graying hair can take on a life of its own, texture-wise. This is out of your control, so you'll need an expert to give you a fantastic haircut when your hair is going gray or white.

Home Hair Color: Drugstore hair color can be extremely tricky to use, especially for hair coloring neophytes. It is particularly difficult to go lighter, so I wouldn't recommend anyone do that at home. The quality and density of the pigments and its ratio to peroxide can only be precisely controlled by a qualified hair colorist who understands the chemistry of mixing color, uniquely, for each client. A good colorist is a bit of an alchemist, if not a magician. A home hair color kit simply can't match a good colorist's skills.

Those who color their hair at home also have problems when the color starts to wash out. Many people erroneously reapply the same (or different) color atop what they already have, and the result is a hair color that's even muddier. In addition, gray hair is notoriously difficult to cover. If you color it yourself at home, you might end up with roots that are one color and the rest of the hair another color.

That said, home hair color can be a lot of fun to play around with if you only want subtle changes and you don't have a lot of gray. The temporary colors that wash out with several shampoos are an ideal way to test out different hues.

Using Hair Products and Tools

Having your hair cut, blown out, and styled at a salon is one of life's sweet pleasures for women, just as a haircut and shave at the barber is for men. But because many women see their time at a hair salon as downtime, they're missing a great opportunity to learn how to style their hair if they don't pay attention to what's being done.

Obviously, you can't blow-dry your hair at home the way a stylist, who's constantly moving all around you, can. Don't be shy about asking what, precisely, is being done during your blow-out. And don't be shy about asking for a style that's easier to replicate at home, depending on how handy you are with the tools you already have.

Hair products have changed tremendously over the years. When I was a child, one of my aunts, my dear aunt Molly whom I loved dearly, wore way too much makeup and used way too much hairspray. As much as I wanted to see her, when I was a little boy I dreaded greeting her because I knew I'd be walking away with gobs of lipstick and sticky remnants of hair spray on my face. She didn't realize just how aging helmet hair can be! Nowadays, fortunately, there is a huge variety of hair products available for all kinds of hair, at drugstore prices.

The best way to find the right hair-care products is to ask your stylist. You need to be blunt about your schedule and how much time you have for styling, and your stylist needs to be blunt about the texture and shape of your hair.

What works well on your sister might not be right for you. Products with a lot of silicone, for instance, might be too dense for those with thin hair, making hair look sticky, but a little bit of mousse can add a lot of volume. Only experimentation, based on your stylist's advice, will lead you to the perfect products for your hair's style and texture.

Many women make the mistake of frying their hair as the heat settings on their blow dryer, flat iron, or curling iron are too high. Yes, you do need a bit of heat, but you don't need to cook your hair! Ask your stylist for recommendations for good home styling products that won't put your hair and scalp at risk.

Bad Hair Days

There are the days where your hair is just a mess, you're running late, and you can't find the blow dryer because your teenage daughter has it stashed under her bed. But you still need to look presentable.

If your hair is long enough to pull back into a sleek ponytail, do that first, as long as the look suits your face shape and features. Accessorize your hair the way you do your outfit. One of the best tricks is to use your own hair as a hair band. Take an elastic hair band and make a ponytail, then from the bottom use a swath of your hair to wrap around the band. Use hairpins to secure it.

You can also get a wardrobe of headbands for a variety of different looks. Or, if you have a deft hand, another option is a clip-on hairpiece so subtle no one would ever guess it's not yours!

STYLE BASICS—MAKEUP

One of the easiest ways to keep your BQ high is with a simple makeup routine that takes just a few minutes in the morning. Once your face is done, you'll be able to refresh your look all day in no more than a minute or two. And as with clothes, once you have a makeup routine that's quick and flattering, you'll leave the house knowing you're always going to look terrific. Creating a subtle yet practical makeup routine is the equivalent of creating your basic clothing wardrobe—and this makeup "uniform" will never let you down.

The goal of this routine is to make you look as if you're not really wearing very much makeup at all. It's the at-home version, in a way, of good plastic surgery. You don't want to look too obvious or too *done*. You simply want to look relaxed and refreshed.

At first glance, it may seem like there are a lot of steps, but Valerie doesn't need more than about five minutes, total, to "get her face on" in the morning, and she never leaves the house without it. So while this makeup routine may take a bit of practice at first, especially when you start to use the proper tools, the more you do it, the quicker and easier it will become.

Think of your makeup routine as the glamorous version of brushing your teeth!

Makeup basics:

- Sheer foundation

- Concealer

- Powder

- Blush

- Eyebrow pencil or shadow

- Mascara

- Lipstick

Optional items:

- Eyeliner

- Eye shadow

Using the Right Tools

The right tools are a necessity, no matter what you're doing. I am very particular about what I use in the operating room, such as special scissors designed for face-lifts, jeweler's forceps, a headlight, and nasal instruments. Good makeup artists are also very particular about their brushes, sponges, foundations, and colors are the tools they need to do their work effectively. So you can't expect to replicate a professional's efforts at home unless you have some of the basic tools at hand.

Valerie keeps her brushes in a cup in the bathroom so they're easily accessible, and she also has a traveling makeup kit with smaller brushes, so she's always prepared in case she needs touchups during the day.

Basic makeup brushes:

- Large, soft brush for powder
- Medium to large soft brush for blush/bronzer
- Foundation sponges
- Lip brush
- Eyebrow brush
- Eye shadow brushes

Powder and blush brushes: Powder and blush brushes are medium to large, round, and fluffy. Ideally, you want natural bristles, as they'll last much longer and give you better coverage.

Foundation sponges: These are available at any good drugstore or beauty supply store, and break apart into triangles. These sponges are inexpensive; even better, by using a foundation sponge instead of your fingers, you will use much less of your costly foundation, so they'll save you money in the long run. Sponges allow you to have more control, and give you the most even coverage with no waste.

To use sponges properly, first wet the sponge lightly, and then squeeze out all the water. You want the sponge only very slightly damp. Then put a small dab of foundation on your hand, and then dip the sponge into it before applying to your face. You'll see an instant difference, with a smoother, more sheer, even finish.

Lip brush: There's nothing more iconic than the sight of a woman putting on her lipstick, tube in hand, so you may be surprised to learn that a lip brush will actually give you a smoother application and better coverage. All you have to do is dip the brush in the color and apply. Look for a small brush with full bristles. This is a very basic item, so don't spend a lot on one. The only real difference is whether the bristles are retractable or if you use a cover.

Eye shadow brushes: The little white-tipped applicators that come with containers of eye shadow are basically useless, so I suggest you throw them out and use small eye shadow brushes instead. Have several on hand for different colors, and always use a slightly fluffier brush for blending. Using soft, natural-bristle brushes is also much easier on tender eye skin and allows the color to be deposited more evenly.

Taking Care of Your Brushes

Brushes must be cleaned regularly, or they'll become repositories for bacteria. Wash them at least every week, depending upon usage, with soap and water, or a bit of shampoo and warm water. Rinse thoroughly and shake them out. Dry them on their sides on a towel. If you dry them upright, water can run down into the wooden handles, which will eventually warp.

Daily Makeup Routine

Now that you are set with the right tools, you can learn this quick seven-step makeup routine that will ensure that you leave the house looking your best every day. At first, this may take some time to get through, but once you learn it and understand the motions, you should be able to put on your face in just a few minutes.

Step 1: Foundation. Don't think of foundation as the thick, cakey formulas that your mom's generation might have slathered on with a trowel, giving them a visible mask. The formulas you can find today are lightweight, non-comedogenic (won't clog your pores), and sheer enough to look natural.

The function of foundation is to even out your skin tone, which is why it's so essential to use a good one as closely matched to your own skin color as possible. There's just no way to look polished and put-together without a smoothing base of foundation on your face— something women with a high BQ take to heart.

When choosing a foundation, remember that everyone's skin is unique, and the only way to find the right foundation is by testing several different brands. Not on your hands or wrists, but on your face.

And you must test foundation in daylight—not in the fluorescent lights of department stores. Ask for a little sample, and then step outside the store and look at the sample with a small hand mirror. You want the foundation to match your own skin as closely as possible. It's easier to find one that's right if you test several samples next to each other. The least visible one is the one you want. In fact, go for the sheerest coverage you can, as this will always look the most natural. If you are fortunate enough to have a fairly even skin tone, use foundation sparingly and only where needed, most often in the T zone area. Less is more!

As foundation is by far the most important item in your makeup kit, you should plan to spend the most on it. The more inexpensive foundations found in drugstores have improved tremendously in recent years, but you need to have a sharp eye and a deft hand to apply it well. The more expensive brands usually have formulations with more "slip," so they go on smoothly and last longer, and they also tend to have more intense pigments in them, particularly yellow (with less pink), so they match more skin tones.

When applying foundation, always blend it down your neck but ever so lightly, as you don't want to overzealously apply a thick layer there. Dab the foundation all the way down to the base of your neck with your sponge, and blend carefully. You'll lower your BQ instantly if there's a noticeable difference between the color of your face and the rest of you! Also, use foundation as a makeup base on your eyelids and lips. This will not only allow the color to last longer, the color will be more true to how it looks in the container or tube.

Step 2: Concealer. Most women need a little concealer, especially as they grow older. Yet concealers are one of those makeup items that can utterly undo a flawlessly made-up face, leaving whitish circles under the eyes or streaks of color around the lips that unwittingly highlight fine lines and wrinkles rather than concealing them.

Choosing a concealer is very similar to choosing a foundation. Make sure you test colors in daylight, and keep testing until you find one that is just a tad lighter than your foundation. As most women with fair to medium skin tend to have a yellowish undertone, look for one that is more peachy than pink. Test as many different brands as necessary for the closest match.

After you put on your foundation, apply a very small dab of concealer with a brush, and blend it carefully. Since concealer is more opaque than foundation, you only need a little bit to be effective. You might want to experiment with different concealer brushes until you feel comfortable blending. Try using a hand mirror, and stand near a window for a good approximation of daylight. Keep blending until there are no streaks.

Remember, concealer should not be used on its own—it's meant to be used in tandem with your foundation.

Step 3: Powder. Like foundation, powder is essential if you want to look polished. Consider it your finisher. It's a must, as it's going to hold everything in place.

Yet many women are afraid to use powder, as they're worried they'll look cakey or fake. Just follow the rule that choosing a powder is not unlike choosing a foundation when it comes to color. You don't want one with too much pink in it or one that's noticeably lighter or darker than your foundation. Yellow undertones help to hide reddish and bluish discolorations. If you use a sheer mineral powder, it should not even be noticeable. Its function is solely to set the foundation you just applied and further even out your skin tone.

Powder should be applied with a large soft brush. Lightly dust the powder evenly across your face and neck—you should only need a very small amount. It's also a good idea to refresh your powder throughout the day. This will keep you looking fresh and get rid of that shine that sometimes appears. Use loose powder at home, and take a compact with pressed powder in your travel makeup bag for later in the day.

Step 4: Blush. Blush is another killer when it comes to BQ scores. Use too much and you can resemble Bozo the Clown. Use too little and you can look washed out and wan. I'd say that far more women overuse rather than underuse blush, and that's because they don't yet have the knack of finding the sweet spot and knowing precisely where to apply it. Blush is meant to give a nice little pop to your palette, so you look vibrant.

Blush should be applied and gently blended with a soft brush to the apple of each cheek. You can find the apple when you smile happily and a little fleshy bit pops out. If you have trouble finding the precise right spot, stand in front of a mirror and feel your cheeks. You'll find the apple, as it's where your cheek bone stops short.

A common mistake for those with round-shaped faces is to think you're creating the illusion of cheekbones by brushing a swipe of color under the cheekbone. This just looks fake. Use just a little blush on the apples of your cheeks instead.

When choosing a blush type and color, there are many things to consider—skin tone, blush color, desired effects. If you're planning to do any contouring, make sure to use a powder blush. While cream blush lasts longer, it's harder to blend, making its use logical only for a quick pop of color.

The color of your blush is very important, as the wrong shade can make you look fake and obviously done up. The most universally flattering blush color is peach-toned. But you can have a blush palette, and play around with different colors. You can also look into scheduling a free consultation with a knowledgeable consultant at a department store makeup counter. The professionals there can help you choose colors if you are feeling overwhelmed by the task.

About Bronzer

Using bronzer can be a great technique to add some color to your face. But don't consider it part of your basic makeup kit. Bronzers tend to have a metallic sheen that can be very appealing in the container, but it is obviously fake color. It's essential to use a very gentle hand when applying bronzer, and many women to tend to go overboard, so they have unsubtle streaks of a color not known to nature in the middle of their face. Not the look you're hoping for!

An easy alternative is a good self-tanner. If you do use one, be sure that your face, neck, and body all end up the same color! Start with the lightest shade and then add on, as the last thing you want to do is look orange.

Step 5: Eyebrows. Eyebrows are fantastically diverse, from Audrey Hepburn and Elizabeth Taylor's famously dark arched brows to Brooke Shields and Sharon Stone's iconic straight brows. Christy Turlington's beautiful thick arch is another example of a gorgeous shape.

Eyebrows can completely change your face, framing your eyes and giving shape to the rest of your features. The results can be astonishing when you have your eyebrows shaped for the first time. Yet if eyebrows aren't shapely, they can easily ruin your whole look. Most women downplay the importance of eyebrows, but a keen eye for shaping in proportion to the rest of your features, along with little bit of grooming, is essential.

Shaping your own brows for the first time is very difficult, so it's worth having them waxed or tweezed professionally. Once the shape is good and set, it's easy to tweeze stray hairs yourself. When you're beginning to tweeze at home, a good trick is to color in your brows with shadow or pencil to the desired shape, and then tweeze the stray hairs that go outside that shape. Once you get used to tweezing, this probably won't be necessary, but it's a good learning tool.

When thinking about brow shape, remember that proportion and moderation are key. Your brow must fit your face. If you have strong features, a strong brow is generally a good idea. If you have delicate features, a thinner brow is called for. Thick or thin, a good brow is a groomed brow. However, there are a few things you should watch out for. Eyebrows that are too thin tend to be both distracting and aging, or too shapeless. Also, one of the worst shapes is to have a thick bulb close to your nose, tapering to a thin line. Try to go for a fairly even eyebrow shape.

Once your eyebrows are shaped, color is the next step. Few women have eyebrow hairs that are all the same color, or with eyebrow color distributed evenly from end to end, so using a shadow or pencil will not only reinforce the shape, but even out the color. You'll be amazed when your brows are evenly colored for the first time!

Pencil is harder to work with, because you can inadvertently create the kind of harsh lines you want to avoid, so until you have a skilled hand, I would recommend an eyebrow shadow. Use your eyebrow shadow and brush to lightly fill in the spaces and even out the color. The key here is *lightly*. After you apply the color with an eyebrow brush with stiff bristles, use a toothbrush to blend it. This step is essential, as it will soften the color and make it look more natural. Doing your brows should take no more than a minute, but the difference in your appearance (and your BQ) is well worth the time.

Most women with light to medium skin tone and eyebrow hair that's brown should use a light to medium brown shadow. Those with darker hair can go for a darker hue. Don't feel you have to match the brow to your hair color exactly.

Step 6: Mascara. Mascara is great stuff. It adds that extra bit of definition and length to your lashes and makes you look more awake.

The color of your mascara is extremely important. Black mascara is strong and dramatic, but can be overpowering for anyone with delicate features or light skin. If black doesn't naturally go with your skin tone, save black for nighttime and use a brown or a brown-black during the day. If you're very light skinned or have red hair and even brown looks unnatural, there is now auburn mascara that will better suit your face. If you can't find it at your local drugstore, you can buy it online.

When applying mascara, apply it fully to each eyelash, one entire eye at a time rather than moving back and forth. This quick break to put mascara on the other eye will give the already applied mascara time to dry. If you apply another coat on top of already dried mascara, it's likely to cake and look unnatural. Using a slight back and forth movement while drawing the mascara brush up your eyelashes will help keep them separated and get color on all sides of your lashes. Remember, adding too much mascara on your lower lashes can look fake, especially if your lower lashes are sparse. Try using mascara only on the outer corners.

You should have to apply mascara only once each day, but be sure to check your makeup every few hours. Mascara can sometimes smudge, giving you a raccoon look that is always unattractive. A few Q-tips in your travel bag will give you all the tools you need to clean up renegade mascara.

Waterproof mascara is wonderful if you're going to the beach or to a wedding where you know you're going to cry, but it's a pain to remove—and you always must remove mascara every night. It can not only break off your lashes but also end up all over your pillow and the rest of your face. Non-waterproof formulas wash off and will streamline your nightly washing routine.

Step 7: Lipstick. Lips are like eyebrows—they're incredibly important for framing your face. But if the color on your lips is too much or too shiny, your BQ will suffer for it.

To apply your lipstick, first put a thin layer of foundation on your lips and lightly dust it with powder. This will create a neutral base that will hold the color longer and allow the color to be true to what you see in the tube. Lip liner, the next step, is important for defining the shape of your lips. First draw an outline around the outer edges your of lips. This barrier defines shape and helps prevent lipstick from working its way off your lips. You should also apply a thin coat of pencil liner all over your lips, and then smudge gently. This will give your lipstick extra staying power throughout the day. The best tone of lip liner to use for your daily routine is one that closely matches the natural color of your lips.

After the lip liner is applied, the next step is to apply your lipstick atop the liner with a lip brush. This will be easier to control. Blend carefully. Then blot. Blotting is the *most* important step of all, as it will remove the excess color and help blend the lipstick with the liner. Your lips will look much more natural, even if you've applied a deep color, and the color will last a lot longer.

If you're in a hurry, you can simply put some lip gloss on top of the liner base. The liner base will still have a bit of color, and the gloss will enhance it. Avoid super-shiny glosses, as they look fake and wear off quickly.

Once you've mastered this technique—foundation base, lip liner on entire lips, smudge, apply lip color with a brush, blot—you will be amazed at quickly you can do it, and how much better your lips look!

A Professional Makeup Consultation

Just as hiring a personal trainer for a few sessions can show you the proper form and most effective way to exercise, having a consultation with a makeup professional can give you useful tips and help you find the best looks, for casual day and more dressy night, for your features and coloring. The best way to learn is to have the makeup artist do half your face, and you do the other half under his or her tutelage.

Department stores with makeup counters offer free makeovers. (But don't feel pressured into buying items you don't need!) Tell the makeup artist what you're looking for. If you feel the need to update your look, ask for a palette that's different from what you typically use. You may be pleasantly surprised by the outcome.

Optional Makeup Routine

Eyeliner. Most eyes benefit from some sort of eyeliner because it makes them better defined. A thin line of black eyeliner is certainly a classic look, but it takes a steady hand and a lot of practice with those tiny brushes to get the line just right. Pencil liners are much easier to use. Remember, blending is key. You don't want the liner itself to be too obvious. And have fun experimenting with different color combinations and textures.

Eye shadow. Mascara is a must, but eye shadow is not. Subtle neutrals are universally flattering and can be unobtrusive yet give your eyes a bit of pop; bolder colors or smoky shadows can give you a sultry look for evening. As there are countless different colors and textures available. The only way to find those you love is to experiment. The look you're going for is subtle and polished, and too much color can actually detract from this.

As with your lips, prepare your eyelids by applying a thin layer of foundation, followed by a light dusting of powder. This will be a base for the color. It will also help even out your skin if it's getting a bit crepey. Then use a small brush with natural bristles to apply the shadow. Dip the brush in the color, and then blot it on a tissue, tap the brush, or blow on it. This will get rid of excess shadow and instantly tone down the color and prevent you from overapplying it.

There are different ways to apply eye color, depending upon the shape of your eyes. A good general rule is to start on the outer part of the upper lid and go into the crease, just under the brow bone. If you want to cover the whole upper lid, be aware that this can create a smoky look, which is generally an evening look. A neat trick if you're not in the mood for shadow but still want a bit of color near your eyes is to use your blush brush and sweep a tiny bit of blush under your brow bone.

Another trick to brighten eyes is to put a dab of light highlighter shadow, such as a cream color or subtle white, into the horizontal "V" outlining the inner corner of your eye and pointing to the bridge of your nose. This area tends to be darker, and this technique can give an instant pop.

Getting Out of a Makeup Rut

It's nearly impossible *not* to get into a makeup rut at some point or another, as it can be downright scary to change your palette. It can also be a way to avoid the fact that you're getting older, and need to make changes in other areas of your life as well. That struck me one day, when a friend of Valerie's was lamenting that she couldn't use her favorite vibrant, shocking pink lipstick anymore, because she'd outgrown it. It was just too bright for her once she hit 50, in the same way as her formerly adorable miniskirts and hip-huggers were no longer age appropriate. Fortunately, she grew just as fond of her new palette (and wardrobe) over time.

If you think it's time for a change, you might want to consider a professional consultation. You don't have to change your entire palette at once, of course. Try a new blush or a different eye shadow. Changes can be very subtle or very dramatic—whatever you're comfortable with. And have fun with it! Try experimenting with a girlfriend to get a second opinion, but always trust your gut before you succumb to someone else's opinion.

After seeing so many patients post-face-lift over the years, I can tell you that hair and makeup do need adjusting when your look has been altered, even subtly. Even without a procedure as dramatic as a face-lift, it's just as crucial to make hair and makeup adjustments with each decade as needed. When done well, you can take years off your appearance.

PART IV

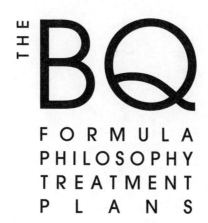

THE **BQ**
FORMULA
PHILOSOPHY
TREATMENT
P L A N S

CHAPTER SEVEN

At-Home Treatment Plans

When you're considering different treatments to enhance or improve your BQ, this is the where you should turn to tackle all issues that haven't been covered in previous chapters. You'll find specific tips for all parts of your face and body—everything that's the least invasive, the least time consuming, the least painful, and the least expensive. These are all treatments that you can do by yourself, at home.

If, however, you have certain genetic traits, such as prominent ears, deep nasolabial fold (the lines between your nose and your lips) or glabellar lines (frown line near your inner eyebrow), or dark circles under your eyes, you will find detailed information about medical procedures in Appendixes B and C.

The following lists are in alphabetical order, and the same format will be followed in Appendixes B and C.

FACE, HEAD, AND NECK

Cheeks—Lack Definition

Treatment: Contouring makeup; haircut.

When You'll See Results: Instantly.

Inside Scoop: Using makeup to contour your cheeks, giving the illusion of cheekbones, takes skill and practice. If you have very round cheeks, it might be worth seeking out a professional makeup artist who can teach you some contouring tricks. It is nearly impossible to figure out how to do this on your own.

Geometric haircuts, where the hair falls against your midface, distracting the eye from your cheeks, are also a possibility.

Chin—Too Prominent

Treatment: Makeup; haircut.

When You'll See Results: Instantly.

Inside Scoop: The way to counterbalance a prominent chin is to enhance the top half of your face with makeup. This means paying particular attention to your eyebrows as well as your eyes. If your eyes are smoky or slightly dramatic, it will pull attention away from your chin. Avoid intense lip color or gloss.

A haircut that also draws the eye away from the chin area can give the illusion of volume in the rest of your face.

Chin—Too Weak

Treatment: Makeup; haircut.

When You'll See Results: Instantly.

Inside Scoop: As with a prominent chin, play up your other features, particularly your eyes, and discuss haircuts with your stylist. Pulling your hair back will accentuate a weak chin, and cuts that fall softly near your chin will make it seem larger.

Ears—Sticking Out

Treatment: Haircut.

When You'll See Results: Instantly.

Inside Scoop: Ponytails and headbands are not likely to be part of your styling tricks, but a haircut that leaves hair covering large ears will do wonders!

Eyes—Bags/Circles Under Lower Lid

Treatment: Concealer; soothing treatments.

When You'll See Results: Instantly.

Inside Scoop: Concealer, properly applied to dark circles, can instantly erase them. Make sure your skin is moisturized first, and then apply foundation, which will even out your skin tone. Then apply concealer with a small brush and blend carefully.

If your under-eye skin tends to be puffy when you wake up or after a long day, try this handy trick. Place a wet but not sopping black tea or chamomile tea bag, or slices of cucumber, on your eyes, and lie down with your eyes closed for a few minutes. They really do work, because the tannins in tea are a natural anti-inflammatory. And the cool cucumber feels good as it reduces swelling and fits on your face.

Eyes—Crepey Skin on Upper Lid

Treatment: Makeup and regular use of eye creams with retinol, vitamin E, and antioxidants, such as Myoxinol (the active antioxidant in my line of face creams).

When You'll See Results: With makeup, instantly; with treatment creams, not before six to eight weeks of regular use. With any treatment cream, do not expect instant results.

Inside Scoop: Eye creams with the above ingredients can reduce very fine lines around the eyes (and the rest of your face), but they must be used daily and results may vary. Don't expect to see any changes for at least six to eight weeks.

Although the eyelid skin is thinner than regular skin and may be more sensitive, fine lines and wrinkles, whether they're on the eyelids or the cheeks, are essentially the same. So you can use your regular moisturizer if you like, although obviously you don't want to get any into your eyes as they can sting badly and cause irritation. The big difference between a regular moisturizer and an eye cream is that products designed for the eye area have been formulated not to cause irritation.

Eyelid skin that needs serious attention can't be treated at home, as these procedures can cause eye irritation or damage.

Always apply a thin layer of foundation on your eyelids prior to using eye shadow, then lightly powder to set the foundation before putting on the color. This will alleviate most of the crepey texture (if you have it) and also conceal any noticeable veins. It will also take some experimentation with different eye shadow textures and formulas to find one that doesn't accentuate any crepey texture. Some women will find that primer actually highlights the texture, so they'll be better off using a powder formulation. Avoid using heavy or brightly colored eyeliner, as this will call attention to your eyelids.

If your eyes are deeply set and the skin is beginning to sag, it might be worth getting makeup lesson, as there are tricks, such as using different shades of highlighter, that will give the illusion of raising your eye bone slightly. Whatever you do, be sure to blend carefully, as seeing streaks of white highlighter under your brow is not a good look! Also be aware that white highlighter should be avoided, as it's way too pale for anyone, no matter how fair, and is actually a very harsh and aging color on your face.

Face—Age Spots

Treatment: Whitening and brightening creams.

When You'll See Results: Six to eight weeks.

How Long It Lasts: For as long as you keep using the products.

Inside Scoop: Freckles might look adorable on a five-year-old's cheeks, but they're still a sign of sun damage. It's important to understand that the pigment system of our skin is a biological necessity. We need it to provide some degree of protection against the damaging effects of the sun's ultraviolet rays.

The color of your skin is determined primarily by the quantity, distribution, and chemistry of the melanin that appears in the outer layer of skin (the epidermis). Melanin is produced by cells within the deeper layer of the epidermis.

As we age, this melanin undergoes changes. Freckles or sun spots, called ephelides or solar lentigo (which are tan or brown maculae with irregular borders on the skin; they're larger than freckles), become more prevalent as the skin overproduces melanin in an effort to protect itself from the sun. Freckles appear on the sun-exposed skin of the face, arms, shoulders, and décolleté. They're most common in childhood and usually disappear during later adulthood. Extensive freckling associated with redheads is an inherited trait, and these freckles will appear in ever-increasing numbers after sun exposure.

Solar lentigo are seen only in adulthood, particularly on those with very fair skin, and they show up on chronically sun-exposed areas, especially the backs of hands, the face, and arms.

Reverse freckles in the form of white dots, called hypo-pigmentation or depigmentation, can also appear; they're caused by sunlight destroying the cells that produce melanin.

Many women notice that their skin is getting blotchy, too. Hyperpigmentation, or areas of deeper pigmentation of the skin, can appear in patches—and it should be no surprise that hyperpigmentation is also a direct result of excessive sun exposure.

Many skin-care companies have launched OTC whitening and brightening creams, usually with hydroquinone as the active ingredient. There is some controversy about hydroquinone's safety, as it is banned in Europe and Japan over fears that it is a potential carcinogen. According to the FDA, hydroquinone is safe and effective—and I believe it is, and is commonly prescribed by many dermatologists in the United States—but if you're worried, look for whitening products that include other bleaching agents, such as kojic acid.

The reason I don't recommend OTC whiteners and brighteners is because bleaching agents, such as hydroquinone, must be used in concentrations strong enough to be effective—and no OTC product is permitted to have that amount of the active ingredients. So you'd be much better off consulting a dermatologist and starting with a prescription-strength product, under medical supervision.

Those with medium to dark skin should never use whitening products without first consulting a dermatologist. Actually, it's always a good idea to see a dermatologist for an annual skin check, to have all spots and moles examined as a precaution against skin cancer. Don't self-diagnose, as you could end up causing more problems in the long run. Ask for advice about which OTC whiteners or brighteners might be right for you and how long you should use them.

You must be hypervigilant about using sunscreen whenever you use lighteners or brighteners, as they make your skin much more susceptible to the sun's powerful rays. If you don't protect your skin, you'll end up getting even more sun spots, which is counterproductive!

Don't forget that you can create a wonderful wardrobe of sunglasses and hats to not only look sensational but to add another layer of protection against the sun.

Face—Blotchy, Dull Skin

Treatment: Exfoliation products; home microdermabrasion kits.

When You'll See Results: Within a few days.

How Long It Lasts: For as long as you keep using the products.

Inside Scoop: As skin ages, the sloughing off of the topmost layer of skin cells, which are actually *dead* skin cells, slows down. This happens to everyone, and explains why skin can lose its luster and become dull and blotchy as you age.

Fortunately, OTC treatments that speed up skin-cell removal work extremely well. Look for exfoliants or home microdermabrasion kits, and try them out till you find one you like. They'll easily remove the dead skin cells and leave your skin looking fresher.

Always follow directions, because with exfoliants, less is definitely more. You can really irritate your skin if you overuse these products. Start out using an exfoliant no more than twice a week, and gradually increase usage as long as there is no irritation or redness.

Face—Deep Grooves (Nasolabial Fold)

Treatment: OTC wrinkle fillers (creams, not injectibles).

When You'll See Results: Immediately.

How Long It Lasts: A few hours, at most.

Inside Scoop: Trying to hide lines between the nose and lips with a thick layer of foundation or concealer is not going to do the trick. Many skin-care companies have wrinkle fillers that temporarily smooth the skin. They work by temporarily plumping up the skin. I'm not a fan, but go ahead and test them in the department store. If you think you see results, and if these results last a few hours, great. If not, you'll need to move on to more invasive treatments such as injectible fillers.

Face—Fine Wrinkles

Treatment: Moisturizers; wrinkle creams.

When You'll See Results: Six to eight weeks.

How Long It Lasts: As long as you keep using the product, but as aging is inevitable, some lines may deepen over time.

Inside Scoop: Using a good moisturizer adds hydration to the topmost layers of your skin, so it will always help with fine lines improving the overall look and texture of your skin.

OTC creams with retinol, vitamin E, and antioxidants are excellent for maintaining the quality of your skin and may help reduce fine lines and wrinkles. The combination of these ingredients seems to work synergistically, so look for this combination for maximum results.

Different products have different ingredients (such as a variety of antioxidants) and in varying concentrations, so if one cream does not seem to be giving you visible results after six to eight weeks, you may want to try another. As with eye creams, if you expect immediate results, you're not going to get them. In fact, many women are impatient, serial moisturizers! They're needlessly wasting their money and exposing their skin to potential irritation because they don't give a new moisturizer the time to do its work effectively.

Once you find a moisturizer that you do like and appears to be doing its job, stick with it. And remember that hype doesn't often match reality, and there are many terrific moisturizers that aren't expensive.

Face—Moderate to Severe Wrinkles

Treatment: Wrinkle treatment creams.

When You'll See Results: Never.

Inside Scoop: I hate to be so blunt, but the fact of the matter is that wrinkle treatment creams for anything other than very fine lines and wrinkles simply do not work. And they will *never* work. There is no miracle in a jar that can treat serious wrinkles, as much as the hyped-up ads in women's magazines might lead you to believe. More invasive treatment, such as injectible fillers, is required.

Because the hype about these OTC wrinkles creams designed to treat medium to deep wrinkles is so pervasive, it's become one of the true danger zones of skin care—the danger being your bank account can disappear while the wrinkles remain.

The best way to treat moderate to severe wrinkles is prevention. Stay out of the sun, so you don't get them in the first place!

Face—Sagging/Wrinkles/Jowls

Treatment: There is no home treatment for sagging skin or jowls and the wrinkles that come with them. See Appendixes B and C.

Forehead—Sagging

Treatment: There is no home treatment for a sagging forehead. See Appendixes B and C.

Forehead—Too High/Prominent

Treatment: Haircut.

When You'll See Results: Immediately.

Inside Scoop: A prominent forehead can easily be disguised with bangs. Avoid center parts or any hairstyles that focus the eye on your forehead.

Headbands can also shift the proportion of your forehead, especially if you have bangs, as they'll make your head appear larger.

Forehead—Wrinkles/Frown Lines

Treatment: Wrinkle creams.

Inside Scoop: See the sections on Face—Fine Wrinkles and Face and Face—Moderate to Severe Wrinkles, above.

Hair—Loss

Treatment: Minoxidil (Rogaine for women); haircut and/or color.

When You'll See Results: Rogaine takes a few weeks to start working. Another product, called Propecia, has been proven to be effective in stopping hair loss in men only, but it has some potential side effects (such as impotence), and it does not work for everyone. Propecia is *not* recommended for women, so you should not use it. With a haircut and color, results are immediate.

How Long It Lasts: For as long as you use it.

Inside Scoop: Hair loss in women is extremely common, but there is so much embarrassment attached to it that many people suffer in silence. Minoxidil is FDA-approved for hair growth in women and men. It's impossible to predict if it will work well for you, but it's worth a try, as it's easily available over the counter, and it has few side effects. But if you are trying to become pregnant or are pregnant already, consult your obstetrician before using Rogaine.

If you don't want to try Rogaine, a good haircut can often disguise hair loss. It may be hard to have either a very short or a very long hairstyle, so be honest about what your hair is like with your stylist, as he or she will already have noticed how much hair has been lost. Adding lots of layers will give depth as well as the illusion of more hair. Don't forget to experiment with hair thickening shampoos, conditioners, and treatment products.

You might also want to think about coloring your hair, as that coats the hair shaft and makes it thicker, so you'll instantly look as if you have more hair. And don't forget about the huge array of wigs, hairpieces, extensions, and weaves that can give you a full head of hair.

Lips—Too Thin

Treatment: Lip plumpers.

When You'll See Results: In a few minutes after application.

How Long It Lasts: A few hours at most.

Inside Scoop: Lip plumpers have gone from 0–60 seemingly overnight. As soon as they appeared on the market, they were huge sellers, even though they sting and may be irritating and painful.

Unlike other products for the face, lip plumpers really do work—but they do so by irritating the lip tissue, which causes temporary swelling. If used frequently over time, the body will eventually adjust and there will be less swelling. But if you become addicted to your lip plumper, as many of my wife's friends have, an unwanted side effect over time is the unwelcome addition of fine vertical lines near your lips. Since the lips are chronically swelling and then shrinking, the skin around them will be affected.

If you can stand the inevitable tingle, lip plumpers are a reliable option for a big night out or for special occasions—but I don't recommend them for regular use as you really don't want to be using any irritant on the tender skin of your lips on a daily basis!

A much better and perfectly harmless alternative is becoming an expert in lining your lips and applying lipstick properly. Take a look at Madonna to see how someone with fairly thin lips still manages to accentuate them into fullness.

Neck—Prominent Muscle (Platysmal Bands)

Treatment: None—see Appendixes B and C.

Inside Scoop: Although the platysmal bands can't be treated with OTC products, you can disguise them with turtlenecks.

Don't forget to moisturize your neck and apply sunscreen every day. The neck is often quite neglected while faces get all the creams and potions, but once there's visible damage, it's very hard to treat without more invasive procedures.

Neck—Sagging/Jowls
Treatment: See Appendixes B and C.

Nose—Botched Nose Job
Treatment: Surgery—see Appendix C.

Nose—Overly Large/Crooked
Treatment: Haircut; makeup.

When You'll See Results: Immediately.

Inside Scoop: Although you can't really minimize a large nose without surgery, you can redirect attention away from it with a stunning haircut and impeccably made-up eyes and lips.

I often discuss the size and shape of noses with patients who think their noses warrant reshaping. I point out the noses of the hugely successful actresses Meryl Streep and Anjelica Huston, as their strong features make them compulsively watchable. Princess Diana also had a large nose—but who noticed it when she blushed and smiled seductively through lowered lashes? Her nose gave her face definition and distinction, and the line of her famous sweeping bangs directed the eye away from the center of her face.

Another great example of a woman with an enormous nose was the magazine editor Diana Vreeland. Although she was the first to admit that she was not a conventionally attractive woman, she still had an exceptionally high BQ because she worked extremely hard at creating a mesmerizing presence and a highly distinctive style. She did admit, inwardly, to massive insecurities, but outwardly she projected a radiant self-assurance, and she stuck to a look that she knew suited her well, with slicked-back black hair, deep crimson lips, and impeccable grooming.

BODY

Breasts—Cancer/Reconstruction

Treatment: Specialized foam prostheses fit in bras (though they can be hot and uncomfortable); reconstructive surgery; see Appendix C.

Breasts—Sagging

Treatment: Surgery—see Appendix C.

Inside Scoop: Although surgery is the only option for sagging, you can help prevent sags or minimize them by always wearing a well-fitting, supportive bra, especially when you're active. Even a size AA cup can eventually sag due to the inevitable breakdown of supportive ligaments in the chest area. It is especially important to wear a sports bra when doing any exercise, especially sports like running or aerobics that involve a lot of bouncing, even if your breasts are small. Breasts will also appear to sag more after a person loses weight. See Appendix D for exercises for the chest.

Breasts—Too Large

Treatment: Minimizing bras.

When You'll See Results: Immediately.

Inside Scoop: Back and shoulder pain due to overly large breasts is very real and can be debilitating. If you have very large breasts solely because you are very overweight, many insurance companies will not agree to pay for breast reduction surgery unless you can show that an attempt was made to lose weight, or that weight loss did not help the situation.

If your breasts have always been large, they can appear disproportionate to the rest of your body once you lose weight or tone up elsewhere. If so, breast reduction surgery might be recommended.

If surgery is not an option, it's heartening to know that technological advances in fabrics and construction have given relief to millions of women suffering from back pain due to large breasts and badly fitting bras, especially as most women have never been properly fitted and have no idea what size they really are.

You might want to try the Butterfly collection at Ashley Stewart, or the Panache D to K line. The Title 9 catalog has dozens of comfortable and supportive sports bras for large breasts, too.

See Appendix D for exercises for the shoulders and back.

Breasts—Too Small

Treatment: Good push-up and/or padded bras; exercise.

When You'll See Results: Immediately.

Inside Scoop: Fortunately for those with small breasts, there are countless bra styles available, with inserts or padding that can push up breasts to create more cleavage and the illusion of larger size.

Posture is also incredibly important. When you stand up straight—and wear a perfectly fitted, supportive bra—your breasts will automatically look bigger.

Stronger pecs cannot increase actual breast size, but they can firm up the surrounding area by toning and sculpting the muscles, giving the illusion of larger breasts.

There are millions of women with gorgeous figures, beauty, and small breasts. (Audrey Hepburn and Keira Knightley come immediately to mind.) It's unfortunate that our society often seems fixated on large breasts, with rail-thin models and actresses getting implants (and lying about it) because they feel they must keep up with the competition.

Breast augmentation is a very personal decision that should be made only after much thought (and realistic expectations). If you are blessed with other assets like sleek long legs and a perky derriere, the BQ philosophy points toward you accenting those traits—and then your cleavage (or lack thereof) will not even be an issue.

See Appendix D for exercises for the chest.

Buttocks—Too Large

Treatment: Spanx; exercise.

When You'll See Results: About four to six weeks.

Inside Scoop: Spanx are the modern equivalent of a girdle, and they really do work at smoothing the hips and buttocks, making you seem firmer and smaller. You also want to wear clothing that fits properly, and isn't too tight. Avoid pants, especially jeans, with large pockets placed squarely on the butt. Fabrics that drape well and skim the area are a much better idea.

But Spanx are only a temporary fix. To make a real difference in the size of your buttocks, you need to exercise. Luckily, as the gluteus muscles are the largest muscle group in your body, they usually respond fairly quickly to exercises targeting them. This is because there's no such thing as "spot toning"; you can't work on only your gluteus muscles, because they're connected to your hip and legs muscles, too. Any exercises for the buttocks will automatically work and strengthen the hips and thighs as well.

See Appendix D for exercises for the buttocks, hips, and thighs.

Buttocks—Too Small

Treatment: Clothing; exercise.

When You'll See Results: Within four to six weeks.

Inside Scoop: Many women have butts that are very small or flat, and they have as much trouble finding clothing that fits well and enhances their lines.

For those with small buttocks, fit is key. Jeans rarely help a flat butt; they'll make it seem even more negligible. You'll probably need a tailor to help, but you can have your pants and skirts altered so that you appear more curvy.

Another tip is that if you reduce the size of your thighs, your buttocks automatically look bigger.

See Appendix D for exercises for the buttocks, hips, and thighs.

Calves/Ankles—Too Large

Treatment: Weight loss (sometimes); surgery; see Appendix C.

Inside Scoop: You can easily camouflage large calves and ankles by wearing pants or long skirts. A midcalf-length skirt paired with boots will also do the trick. Look for boots that have extra width in the calf area.

Excess Skin—Fat Deposits in Specific Areas

Treatment: Exercise—sometimes.

When You'll See Results: Within four to six weeks.

Inside Scoop: As you know by now, liposuction, especially in the thigh area, is *not* a weight-loss tool, and it's often not needed—toning is. I won't consider performing liposuction unless a vigorous exercise and weight-loss program has been ongoing for at least six weeks. Some women do have genetically determined fat deposits that won't go away no matter how much they exercise, and they will be the ideal candidates for liposuction.

See Appendix D for exercises for the buttocks, hips, and thighs.

Excess Skin—Sagging Skin in Midsection

Treatment: Exercise.

When You'll See Results: Within four to six weeks.

Inside Scoop: The best way to work on your belly area is with cardiovascular exercise, crunches, and diet modification.

If you're not yet a regular exerciser, start small. Walk more. Gradually ramp up your strength and endurance.

Even if you don't have any sagging skin in your middle, doing exercises to strengthen your core is an excellent idea for all women, no matter your size or age. A strong core will add muscle, which will increase your metabolism and help you burn more calories. It will also improve your posture.

That said, stretched skin in the lower abdomen area, due to pregnancy or after a significant weight loss, cannot be corrected by exercise alone; surgical excision is needed. However, the surgery will be that much more effective if exercise has already started to tone the area.

See Appendix D for exercises for the abdominals and core.

Excess Skin—Weight Loss

Treatment: Clothing; exercise.

When You'll See Results: Four weeks.

Inside Scoop: Those who've lost a tremendous amount of weight often find their BQ hindered by leftover rolls of excess skin. Although clothing that fits, especially blouses or sweaters with long sleeves, will help camouflage the skin during the day, it still needs to be dealt with. Surgery is usually the only option to remove excess skin.

That said, I once had a patient who had lost more than 100 pounds through diet and exercise, and who came to me for a thigh lift. To keep her weight down, she'd become an avid and accomplished Latin dancer. She had excellent muscle tone, but was hindered by the excess skin that remained on her thighs, which affected how she danced. I was astonished at how flat she'd gotten her stomach area, as this is usually one place where excess skin is almost impossible to tone without surgery. The moral of the story is that dance had strengthened her core so well that she only needed surgery on her thighs.

She also had toned up her arms. Strong triceps will help firm up excess skin in the upper arms of all women—this is the area that starts to sag noticeably with age, giving you the dreaded jiggle when you wave.

See Appendix D for exercises for the arms.

Hands—Crepey/Thin/Mottled Skin

Treatment: Whitening products; see Face—Age Spots, above.

Inside Scoop: Too bad gloves are considered so last century, as back then, women (other than farm or factory workers) would never leave the house without their hands covered. Sadly, hands are often neglected until damage to thin and delicate skin is noticeable.

Unless you're fashion-forward enough to flaunt a fabulous glove collection, even in the summer, never fail to slather on the sunscreen, keep a good hand cream nearby during the day, and reapply it often. Having regular manicures will also help you pay attention to your hands.

BOGUS TREATMENTS

There are so many bogus treatments for faces and bodies that I constantly marvel at how otherwise educated consumers fall for them.

It's actually very simple to figure out what works and what's hype. I say, "Show me the science." I don't want to know about a treatment that "may" work for a "few weeks"—I want to see proof that effects are not only long-lasting, but also reproducible. In other words, if the science shows that something is effective, the results can be repeated, over and over again, and be identical every single time. I know that when I inject Botox, for example, it is going to paralyze the muscles as intended for nearly all patients (there is an extremely small amount of people for whom it just doesn't work). I know that when I use a laser to target pigmentation, it is going to zap it away.

So while it's perfectly fine to be given a window of time when you ask how long a procedure lasts, if your physician or surgeon appears to be waffling, you should press for an explanation. For instance, if a procedure is very new and you're being told that results always vary considerably, ask why. There's no reason for you to be a guinea pig for as-yet-unproven treatments. Chances are that if it sounds too good to be true, it is! Do not fall for the argument that goes: *It can't hurt, so why not try it!* It just may hurt you—physically, and in the pocketbook!

Bear in mind that if there really were a cure for a tough condition to fix, such as cellulite, you would know about it right away. Every single dermatologist, plastic surgeon, and many other physicians would be offering this treatment!

Some of the most egregious examples of what I consider to be bogus treatments are: acupuncture face-lifts, cellulite creams, electrostimulation (machines that attach to your face and then give out mild electrical currents to allegedly stop skin from sagging by bulking up the facial muscles, or machines that hook up to your abdominal muscles and then claim that the mild shocks will tone these muscles), endermologie (a course of treatment with rollers and suction providing deep massage that allegedly removes cellulite), leeches (yes, those blood-sucking creatures, which do not improve your skin), mesotherapy (subcutaneous injections of vitamins, minerals, amino acids, and/or homeopathic ingredients to allegedly remove cellulite, fat, and wrinkles, which is even more worrying to me as long-term metabolic studies to prove their safety have not been done), and oxygen facials (breathing in oxygen is a necessity; it does nothing to your skin).

CHAPTER EIGHT

Steps to Raise Your BQ—Personal Plans

The beauty of the BQ Formula is that it's not only a lifestyle change but also a plan that can be tailored to specific and immediate goals. Raising your BQ doesn't have to involve radical changes. It can, in fact, be done quickly and easily once you have a good idea of your best attributes and know how to accentuate them.

Whether you have only a few days to prepare for a job interview or six months to get ready for a wedding or reunion or family event, here are some suggestion to help you draw up a plan to raise your BQ before the big day.

IF YOU HAVE FOUR HOURS

What happens if you're given an invitation to an important meeting or event, whether a business function or a surprise date with a new beau, and you have only a short time to get ready? Mustering all your BQ skills will be a breeze once you've mastered the basics. You'll have the confidence to go out knowing that you're looking your best, so you can concentrate on enjoying yourself rather than worrying about how your hair looks or whether your outfit best accentuates your figure.

Clothing

Running to the department store on short notice is a recipe for disaster, because if you're anxiously trying to find something special, you're likely to be too frazzled to use your best judgment. You might end up with an outfit that really doesn't suit you or is way over your budget. It's always best to stick to the several favorites you should already have in your closet—staples that you know flatter you, are comfortable, fit well, and have garnered compliments in the past. Note that the most important element on this list is *fit*. A vintage dress you got at a garage sale that fits you impeccably will always look better than the newest, most trendy dress that does little to highlight your curves.

As for color, black is tried and true and always slimming, but if your favorite outfit is colorful, then go for it. Just remember to accentuate your positives and/or hide your negatives; don't wear a long skirt if you have nice legs, or cover up your décolleté if you have nice cleavage!

Makeup

As with clothing, don't experiment with a new look unless you have time to dash to a makeup counter and have a pro do your face (a trick many of my patients use). Less is more. Stick to your regular makeup routine and colors.

If, and only if, you are already experienced at using self-tanner, then you could try a light application as early as possible before your event, especially on your legs if you're not planning to wear pantyhose. But never try a new product or you might show up looking streaked and orange.

Make sure your hands and nails are well groomed. If you have time, try to get a manicure with a neutral color, or touch up your nails yourself to avoid having to hide your hands during those all-important introductions when handshakes are required.

Hair

You might have guessed by now—this is not the time to experiment with a new hairstyle either. Stick to what makes you look good. Don't panic if your hair isn't perfectly clean as slightly dirty hair is actually easier to style.

If at all feasible, though, have your hair blown out professionally. If your hair is on the short side, a blow-out doesn't take long but you will look fresh and polished. It's a great tool to make you feel confident.

Diet and Exercise

Obviously, with only four hours, you don't have time to do a lot in the diet and exercise area. Many people think that not eating will help them appear slimmer, but in reality this doesn't work. Don't starve yourself, even for a few hours. It won't make you look any better, and it makes it hard to enjoy yourself if your stomach is grumbling.

If you have time, even ten minutes, try to do a light workout to relieve stress and get your blood flowing for an automatic energy boost. You might not have time to really get sweaty, but you can still try to go for a brisk walk, and do some exercises with hand weights, especially for your arms.

Mind-set/Ego Boost

Choose three positive recent memories that fit the situation you're preparing for, then hit the mental rewind button so you can remind yourself of your ability to manage any new situation.

Keep a flattering photo of yourself handy to remind you of how good you really look.

Do a few minutes of conscious breathing in a quiet space to clear your head.

IF YOU HAVE FOUR DAYS

While four hours gives you practically no time to make any changes in preparation for an event, four days should be more than enough time for you to be able to prepare in earnest. You may not be able to lose weight or fix any major problems, but you will have time to experiment and possibly find something new that will up your BQ. Also simply knowing that you're ready will boost your confidence and automatically raise your BQ.

Clothing

Do you really need a new outfit? You probably don't. Try shopping in your closet for a new outfit that you've forgotten. Experiment with new combinations of the tried and true. Just make sure that what you wear fits perfectly. If not, see if a local tailor or dry cleaner can do a quick fix. Have your outfit pressed professionally, too.

If you actually do need a new outfit, four days gives you enough time to find something. Don't try an entirely new style, but a variation on what you know looks good can be found. Try to go shopping on the first or second day of your preparation time. This will give you the chance to run a new outfit by a friend or loved one for a second opinion. It will also allow you time to try it on again at home and get comfortable in it. Being uncomfortable really detracts from your BQ, as you will constantly be fidgeting and self-conscious.

Makeup

This is another area where a few days gives you time to play around with new colors and textures. Wear them out to work or with friends before your four days are up, so you can be sure you like the look. Ask your friends for advice. You can always go back to your regular look if you're not crazy about your experimentation.

If you haven't yet perfected your makeup routine, particularly with your eyebrows, now is the time to practice to get it perfect. You also have enough time to schedule a professional brow shaping if you need one.

Hair

With the time you have, you should be able to get a last-minute hair appointment if you need to touch up your roots or get a trim. Do not make any dramatic changes, as you won't have time to get comfortable with a new look. Also book a blow-out.

Diet and Exercise

While you will have time to make some changes, what you can accomplish are very short-term goals. Do not even consider going on any radical diets, such as juice fasts or "cleanses" or drastic calorie cutting. These can disrupt your blood sugar balance, making you tired and irritable. However, you can decrease salt, which often causes bloating; decrease sugar, which gives you a temporary energy burst followed by a deep crash (and cravings for more sugar); decrease caffeine, which is a stimulant and can disrupt sleep; and decrease alcohol consumption, which adds junk calories while also disrupting sleep. Reducing these items, for even four days, can make a big difference in your energy level and how you look. Eat sensibly, adding lots of fruits and vegetables to your diet if you don't eat them already.

Try to do at least one to two light cardio workouts to relieve stress and get your blood flowing. Add a round of the exercises from Appendix D. Although you won't notice a difference in only four days, you will feel a lot better.

Mind-set/Ego Boost

Sit down with a trusted friend and ask for kind criticism to remind you of any bad habits or nervous gestures. Do you tend to talk too much about old boyfriends when you go on dates? Do you unconsciously twiddle your hair or bite your nails? Is your grooming impeccable? For instance, Valerie has a friend who has short eyelashes on her lower lid, but this woman loves thick black mascara so much that she overdoes it. An hour later, she has raccoon eyes and looks tired and unprofessional—and unfortunately is judged as such. All she had to do to improve her BQ was change her mascara to a lighter shade and apply it a bit more judiciously.

IF YOU HAVE FOUR WEEKS

If summer's approaching and you've been invited out to the beach—yet you've been so busy at work that you haven't paid much attention to your BQ and are worried about how you'll look—what can you do in a month? A lot!

With four weeks for preparation, this is an ideal time to take the BQ Quiz again, select one or two particular areas of concern that have been pointed out by your answers, and get to work. This will be easier if you choose two that go hand in hand, such as diet and exercise or hair and makeup. Having a goal and a date to achieve it by ought to give you the incentive to stick with the plan. Keep your expectations realistic and your enthusiasm up!

Clothing

Four weeks gives you plenty of time to experiment with a new style. If you've been wanting to step up your fashion or simply make a change, go for it. But make sure to start the process during the first week of preparation. This will allow you time to perfect your new look and become entirely comfortable with the new you.

When planning your clothing for an event four weeks out, certainly don't pick out an outfit in week one. Since you have time to watch your diet and exercise regularly, you may lose enough weight during these four weeks that the outfit you chose won't fit properly, which can be very disappointing if you purchase something new and wonderful in the wrong size. It's better to set aside time to choose an outfit about four to five days before the big event—and certainly don't wait until the last minute to try it on. Clear your calendar for that shopping time far in advance. You may also want to scout stores in advance if you have the time, or ask salespeople for recommendations. You don't want a frantic last-minute shopping expedition, which is when it's all too easy to make the wrong decision about an emergency outfit.

Makeup

If you would like to change your look, book an appointment with a professional makeup artist during week one or two. If you do a makeover at the cosmetic counter at a local department store, it's usually free. Discuss why you want a particular look and what products you already own in that color scheme. Ask the makeup artist to do only one side first and try to replicate the look on the other side, if possible. If not, and if you like the look, practice it at home until you've mastered it. You could even try out a couple of new looks, but remember that getting used to a new palette or formulation can take several weeks, so make sure you start practicing in the first two weeks.

Still, bear in mind that makeup artists at the cosmetic counter do need to sell products. Don't allow yourself to be pressured to buy anything that you're not completely convinced is "you." You might want to take a trusted friend along for advice.

Hair

Should you change your hairstyle or color? A fabulous new haircut can be a tremendous confidence builder, and four weeks should give you ample time to figure out which new hairstyling products to use and learn to work with a new cut. Still, with only four weeks, this is not the time for a complete overhaul. Err on the side of caution and choose a style or color that will let you return to your previous look if needed. Haircuts usually need a few days to settle in, and you will also need a bit of time to get used to seeing a new you each time you look in the mirror.

If you want to try a color change in your four weeks, your best option is to go to a salon based on solid word-of-mouth recommendations and discuss your options, and how to reverse any changes in case you're unhappy with them. If you can't afford to do this, you can try an at-home option. At the beginning of the four weeks, try out a non-permanent option. If you are unhappy with the results, you can be certain that it will have worn off before your big event. If you like the color, you can feel safe to reapply it as the time draws closer.

Diet and Exercise

Choose a diet that can help you lose up to two pounds per week, which is a healthy and realistic goal. Avoid any diet that promises more—you'll only be losing water weight, and once you start eating normally again the pounds can quickly pile back on, and then some. Try to significantly cut down on sugar and salt, as this minimizes bloating.

Find the time and determination to add a cardio and hand-weight routine into your four weeks, and stick to it. Map out a schedule that will allow you to do two to three days of at least 30–45 minutes of cardio, as well as two days of weight training for 30–45 minutes each week. If you think this goal is going to be too tough, remember, that you're only going to be doing it for four short weeks of your time. You *can* do it!

Start slow, and don't push yourself in an attempt to see quicker results, as you'll set yourself up for the possibility of injuries or burnout. Hopefully, you'll start to see some real results and, more important, improve your health and your stamina—and find the incentive to incorporate regular workouts into your life—even after your four weeks are up.

Mind-set/Ego Boost

Make a list of all the things you need to do before the big day. Check each off as you finish the task. This tiny little gesture is extremely satisfying!

Don't forget to reward yourself for all your hard work—which means considering a bit of shopping to buy yourself something that looks great. Stick to your budget so you don't end up criticizing yourself for overspending.

Find a fairly recent photo of yourself in which you know you look sensational, and look at it whenever you might be feeling frustrated or having a bad day. It'll be a good reminder of how high your BQ is, and how it will be high again.

Keep a good friend or family member in the loop to help you keep going and to reassure you that your hard work is paying off. Continue to remind yourself that this is only a four-week process. Sure, you will see some improvement, but you still need to be realistic about expectations. There is no magic transformative bullet—but your determination to succeed will always be more potent than a fad diet or unrealistic and unsustainable crash workout plan. And you're only at the beginning of your BQ journey.

IF YOU HAVE FOUR MONTHS

Four months is more than enough time for a subtle yet total BQ overhaul, particularly if you're planning for an important life event, such as a wedding, reunion, job change, or move.

With this amount of time, there should be no reason why you can't achieve your goals (unless, of course, your expectations are unrealistic). As with the four-week plan, retake the BQ Quiz, then draw up a checklist of your goals and devise an action plan. You should be able to remain motivated so you can have a profound influence on several areas you want to change.

Again, try to work in pairs: diet and exercise, hair and makeup, clothing and diet, for example. If you have the time, feel free to choose several pairs of options. Or, concentrate on diet and exercise for the first two months, and then move into maintenance mode on them and start working on your hair and makeup during the next two months. The more you work out and watch your diet, the easier it is to become used to your new routine and modify it according to your schedule.

You might also want to take a full-length photo of yourself in a bathing suit or bra and panties. Put it away and don't look at it. At the end of four months, take another photo in the same position wearing the same bathing suit. You will be amazed at the progress you have made.

This is a common practice for me with my surgical patients. I always take a pre-op photo. People forget what they looked like prior to the surgery, and it's cause for happy amazement when they look back at themselves months later. It's a surprisingly effective way to critically view and assess all your improvements, and then move on to what other work might need to be done.

Clothing

It's now time to get tough and rework your closet and wardrobe. If you don't have the willpower to do it on your own, invite some friends over and have a closet-clearing party. You can even have a clothes swap, where you and your friends pile up all unwanted clothing and then pick and choose what might look good on you. When that's over, donate or give away all the clothing that you no longer wear or that no longer fits well, especially if you've lost weight and reshaped your body. Getting rid of your larger-sized clothing can be extremely satisfying!

You also have plenty of time to experiment with different styles and colors, and may be able to wait for end-of-season sales in your area. Scan the fashion magazines or online shopping sites, and see what catches your eye that potentially and realistically will work for your figure as well as your budget.

If you plan to lose weight or tone up, don't make any major investments in clothing until you start to see real results, which will probably be after at least two to two and a half months.

Makeup

Find your inimitable style and perfect its application so it becomes second nature. You should now be expert at getting your everyday daytime routine done in less than ten minutes. Doing your evening makeup will take a few more minutes, as you'll usually be doing a more intense look, but you should still be more comfortable with the routine and able to do it flawlessly.

For day or evening, experiment with different eye shadows. Play around with them and have fun! You can have a makeup wardrobe as easily as you have a clothing or shoe wardrobe—that's the fun of it! For a special event, you can even work with individual false eyelashes or a full strip lash. Just make sure the look is more Jennifer Lopez and not Liza Minnelli in *Cabaret*!

Hair

You'll have plenty of time to play around and undo any damage should you get a cut or color change that you don't like, so go for it. Book an appointment with a hairstylist or colorist in the first month, so you can get used to anything new. Be sure to make an appointment for a trim and/or color touch-up close to the end of the fourth month or as needed.

Four months also gives you a relaxed amount of time to learn to work with your own hair, so you can rely less on a pro. A special function can warrant a trip to the hairdresser, but for a dinner out or a party, you should now be able to handle the duties yourself.

Diet and Exercise

Major changes can be made in your shape as well as your health, once you're eating a nutritious diet and exercising regularly. Some may need to lose a lot of weight; some may need to gain it. Hopefully, the benefits you'll be seeing and feeling will help you stick to the plan—and make it one that will last a lifetime.

I urge you to consult a registered dietician, who can help you draw up a realistic and doable weight-loss plan. Stick to it and stay committed. Carve out the time to do cardio and weight training for at least four days a week, and keep a workout log. Review it at the end of each month to monitor your progress.

An eating log (no cheating!) can also be a tremendous help for you to see what you're eating and drinking (liquids are often the source of many hidden calories) and why you chose to ate what you did at that particular time. If you're losing weight, you can consult the log to see what is working; conversely, if you're not making progress, it can help you try to understand why.

Mind-set/Ego Boost

Make a realistic list of goals that you wish to accomplish in four months. List every possible change you hope to make. You might not be able to attain all of these goals, but you will certainly attain more than a few.

After four months, evaluate how you did. Make a new list of all the things you changed in your life and your appearance. Then make another still-to-do list. However long or short these lists are, do not become frustrated; changing your BQ is, and always will be, a work in progress. So you should be extremely proud of all your hard work. Be sure to reinforce your accomplishments with self-praise. This is not narcissism—this is simple acknowledgment of a job well done.

Conclusion

Over the many months it took to write this book, I realized how much I have learned about my notions of beauty and self-presentation, and how happy I was to be able to share the countless tips I've gleaned over the years and have also been given from patients and colleagues.

When I was writing, I realized that the initial impetus for *The BQ Formula* went back many years, to the Hippocratic Oath I took when I became a doctor: "First, do no harm." It meant, *What can I do for my patients to help them the most?*

I spent the bulk of my early surgical career doing reconstructive surgery on patients who'd been injured in accidents or battling cancer. This training was incredibly useful as my practice gradually transformed itself to primarily aesthetic surgery. I gained the proper perspective in treating my cosmetic patients from my experiences dealing with the reconstructive patients, especially since accentuating the positives is so much more important for patients who have made it through cancer or who've been injured in an accident. I learned to understand where to draw the line when patient expectations appeared unrealistic.

And then I realized that it meant that not only should I be the most skillful surgeon possible, but that I should also be equally skillful at saying no to those who thought they needed plastic surgery when they didn't. What they needed instead was concrete advice about how to enhance their good points and downplay the bad. To own their beauty without surgery, if possible.

I also wrote this book in homage to my wonderful father, an old-school physician who still made house calls when he was in his eighties and loved his job more than anything (except his family). His motto was, "What can I do to take care of the patients who need me?" He had plenty of patients who didn't have physical ailments, but they still needed him. He made them all feel better. He also taught me humility, and reminded me that our profession is not perfect and that sometimes our patients get better in spite of us!

It is my hope that you will see *The BQ Formula* as a book version of a private consultation with me. That it will help you find your inner and outer beauty, and that you will feel as good about yourself as my father's patients did after he looked them in the eye, smiled, and told them they looked fabulous.

What Medical Procedures Can Do for You, and How to Find the Best Plastic Surgeon for Your Needs

If you're reading this section, I have no doubt that you've exhausted all the options in the previous chapters.

As you saw in the Genetic Destiny section of the BQ Quiz, some people are born with conditions that cannot be self-treated, which makes them ideal candidates for surgical corrections. This list includes those with dark under-eye circles; sagging eyelids, giving a sleepy look; a prominent nose, particularly if coupled with a weak chin or breathing difficulties; lines and wrinkles that make a face look perpetually tired or angry; breasts that are too large or that sag after breastfeeding; fleshy areas that remain in different parts of the body despite vigorous and regular exercise; excess skin after significant weight loss; and any reconstruction after an accident or treatment for an illness.

Before you decide to move ahead with medical treatment, read on, as there are many extremely important issues to consider beforehand.

REALISTIC EXPECTATIONS ABOUT PLASTIC SURGERY AND OTHER TREATMENTS

Many of the patients who come to see me have unrealistic expectations about what plastic surgery can do for them. If someone comes in and announces that she's envious of So-and-so's nose or So-and-so's breasts and wants the exact same thing, this is a clear sign that this person hasn't realistically looked at the situation. So-and-so's breasts might be right for her body size and shape, but they may not be right for the prospective patient.

You have to take a realistic look at your body, and accept that you can't change it entirely to look like someone else's. You cannot change all parts of your genetic destiny with surgery, so it's better to learn to accept much of yourself and change things that can actually be considered flaws. But you must change them in proportion!

Another warning sign that someone may not have realistic expectations is appearance obsession. If a new patient is obsessed with one particular area of the body—to the point of measuring it down to the millimeter and scouring Websites for information about the alleged deformity, she may be in the throes of a psychological condition called body dysmorphic disorder. In this case, surgery is an unrealistic cure; in fact, it can make the situation worse. Body dysmorphic disorder warrants immediate attention from a competent, licensed therapist, to get to the core of the emotional issues leading to this obsession.

In both of these instances, the patient has unrealistic expectations about what surgery can do for her. And in both instances, surgery should not be performed. Without being fully aware and accepting what surgery can actually do for you, you will certainly be disappointed in the outcome of any procedure.

Now let's take a look at the top ten myths about plastic surgery. Addressing these myths will help dispel any unrealistic expectations.

Myth #1: After the Procedure, I'll Look 20 Years Younger

In reality, if your procedure goes the way it should, you should look better. You'll look well rested. And hopefully you'll still look like *you*! But you won't look 20 years younger. Plastic surgery can only do so much for you, and this is one of those instances where unrealistic expectations will just lead to disappointment.

Myth #2: I Won't Have a Scar

An inescapable fact of physiology is that if the skin is cut, with either a scalpel or laser, a scar will form. Obviously a good plastic surgeon will do their utmost to leave minimal or completely unobtrusive scarring, but if anyone tells you that you won't see a trace of the procedure, the only cutting you should be doing is of their phone numbers out of your life.

Myth #3: The Newest Procedures Are Always the Best Procedures

Many allegedly sensational and hotly hyped procedures fizzle fast. It's awfully enticing to read about the Next New Thing in a glossy magazine and hope that whatever's being gushed about might help you. If you immediately make an appointment, without doing any research, you could be sorely disappointed or worse. Research will help you know if the Next New Thing is truly a legitimate technique.

You need to get a number of questions answered before you get on the operating table. For example: How new is this procedure? Was the research peer reviewed (studied by other physician specialists to be certain that it is safe and works)? Are there any other doctors or surgeons doing it? If not, why not? Are the results proven and reproducible?

If a doctor tells you he's the only one doing this new procedure, it may be not because the procedure is so fantastic, but instead because he's being paid a fortune by the manufacturer to test it out. You should also ask for copies of any studies associated with a new procedure. The language might be a bit dense, but you'll be smart enough to figure it out.

Now, I love women's magazines and my wife does, too. But I know enough to be skeptical about claims that say "This treatment will get rid of cellulite once and for all!" or, "I lost an amazing amount of weight plus firmed up my belly after I used this!" or, "I look ten years younger after one lunchtime procedure!"

What many readers don't know is that the Next New Thing is likely to be backed by a very prestigious marketing and public-relations machine whose function it is to sell the products they've been hired to pitch. Or that editors are often given freebies in the form of products or treatments in exchange for a prominent plug in the magazine. Or that advertisers who shell out big bucks for upfront placement in magazines expect a bit of the quid pro quo.

This should not surprise anyone. Advertising is what keeps magazines afloat—not subscribers. And, of course, advertising as well as articles are often tremendously useful, since they show consumers what products or treatments are out there in the marketplace. But you have to read more about them and do your own research so you can make better informed decisions.

Simply bear in mind that the media jumps all over the Next New Thing and pushes it like crazy until the next Next New Thing comes along. Don't fall for the hype! You don't need to pay large sums of money to be a guinea pig for an untested procedure.

Myth #4: Any M.D. Can Do These Procedures

Not long ago, my cousin asked me for my opinion—her gynecologist had told her that he was now doing laser treatments, and he suggested that she have the sun damage on her fair skin treated by him, in his office. What did I think she should do?

I said, "Well, there are two things you can say. One is that you ran this idea by your cousin, a board-certified plastic surgeon, and he doesn't think it's such a good idea. Or you can say, 'Wow, what a wonderful idea. I'm going to go to my dermatologist for my next pelvic exam.' "

My cousin laughed—she got the message. But a lot of people don't. And they might suffer needlessly as a result.

While anyone with a medical license can legally perform surgical procedures in his or her private offices, that doesn't mean he or she *should* perform them! Would you trust your podiatrist to operate on your heart? Or your gynecologist to operate on your brain?

I find it unbelievable how many gynecologists, podiatrists, and other M.D.s are turning over a large portion of their practices to aesthetic or "anti-aging" procedures. These aren't easy procedures to do. To be done well, they take years of training, expertise, and most of all a specific kind of "eye" to understand how best to work on a face or body.

Plastic surgery should *only* be performed by plastic surgeons. Period. That's what I firmly believe, after all my years of training and practicing. I'm not saying that to add to my patient load; I'm saying it because every person deserves to have the best possible treatment performed by the most skillful practitioner.

Take liposuction, for example. To do it well requires skill and experience. Take out too much fat at once, and you can be left with dimples, pockets, or muscle damage—or you could conceivably die when your body goes into shock from fluid loss if large amounts of fat are removed without proper fluid management afterward. The dangers can't be downplayed, but lots of doctors take a weekend training course and then advertise their newest procedure, at enticing prices.

If you don't want to see a plastic surgeon for noninvasive procedures, choose a dermatologist who is certified by the American Board of Dermatology and who has years of experience handling injectibles and/or lasers for a wide variety of patients with different skin tones and conditions. Skin is, after all, a dermatologist's specialty. Many cosmetic dermatologists are as skilled as surgeons with the use of injectibles, such as Botox and fillers like Restylane. They treat thousands of patients each year and have a sculptor's eye, as a good surgeon will. They attend conferences and consult with their colleagues and are up to date on new techniques and products. And their medical training will stand them in good stead should there be any complications warranting prescriptions of antibiotics, or further treatment.

But a dermatologist is still not a surgeon, with a surgeon's years of training. Choose carefully; the face and body you save is your own. Naturally, this is merely *my* opinion, but it is based on years of experience dealing with the many complications caused by other "specialists" *not* sticking to *their* specialty.

Myth #5: Everyone Can Benefit from Plastic Surgery

This myth is vital to discuss, especially as it's one that plastic surgeons are often loath to talk about with their patients. But some patients are just not good candidates for a particular plastic surgery procedure.

I have two primary reasons for turning away a patient: psychological and physical.

A psychological reason usually emerges during our first consultation. If, when I ask, a patient tells me she's unhappy with the tip of her nose because it's drooping, I can work with that. But, if she says, "Do whatever it takes to make me look beautiful," there may be underlying issues that a scalpel cannot fix.

I would say that I turn away 15 to 20 percent of patients who are simply not good aesthetic surgery candidates, who will never be happy with my surgery, no matter how good the result. What they really need to do is to work with a competent therapist, who can help them understand and manage the underlying emotional issues leading them to think that something as radical as an operation will automatically make them happy or beautiful.

A physical reason usually has to do with a patient's weight, smoking, or other preexisting medical conditions. For that reason, we have a very detailed intake sheet that my staff and I meticulously check off, to ensure that all medical conditions and medications are listed. We need to know about all previous surgeries and current medications because these factors will affect the current surgery. The information provided may make us realize that surgery would actually be unsafe.

Sometimes I know the patient would have good results, but I still won't perform the surgery. If weight is the issue, it's unhealthy to have surgery from a strictly medical point of view. Instead, I might recommend noninvasive procedures like injectible fillers that don't require anesthesia or have a huge risk of infection.

Unfortunately, these less-than-healthy patients are often not hard to sway, and they're still able to find a surgeon who will inform them of these risks yet perform the surgery anyway, putting that patient at grave risk for complications or even death.

Myth #6: Breast Implants Are for Everyone

Breast augmentation surgery can be satisfying and rewarding, but it's not for everyone. The decision to have implants placed in your body should not be taken lightly, especially as anyone who gets implants needs to know that the first operation will not be the last operation. Breast implants don't last for a lifetime, which I discuss in more depth in Appendix C.

There are also plenty of misconceptions about what breast surgery can do for you. If you're dealing with some serious sagging, implants will provide some lift, but, often, adding more will not lift you up *enough*—a breast lift may also be needed.

Myth #7: All Lasers Work the Same Way and Are Perfectly Safe

Patients often confront me, aghast that I'm still using a scalpel instead of a laser on certain procedures. They don't understand that lasers are not toys, and in unskilled hands, you can end up with huge splotches all over your face, permanent scarring, or second-degree burns.

There are many different kinds of lasers, each with different functions: some are designed to remove hair or tattoos or birthmarks, others tackle wrinkles or tighten skin. A lot of training is imperative, particularly if you have darker skin tones that necessitate careful calibration of the laser. It is a very risky endeavor to go to a cut-price salon with little medical supervision and a barely competent employee wielding a device that can do serious damage.

Myth #8: An "Extreme Makeover" Will Make Me Extremely Happy

Sometimes, having an extreme makeover can have extremely gratifying results—but only if all the circumstances are right. If you're in very experienced hands, and if you're in terrific shape, and if your condition warrants it, having more than one procedure done at one sitting, or in a fairly small window of time, can be okay and at fairly low risk to your health, although your recovery might be quite painful. But for many patients, it can be not only be too much but also extremely dangerous.

It's often much better and safer to stagger several smaller procedures over appropriate intervals and see how well you heal and how good you look when all the swelling has gone down (which can take months, depending on the work done), rather than endure the potential for disaster any extreme operation brings to the table. If your surgeon doesn't recommend performing the procedures you want at the same time, listen carefully and heed that advice!

Myth #9: The More I Pay, the Better the Procedure

Higher fees actually don't mean higher skills from your surgeon or a safer procedure. One of the best breast surgeons I know has very low fees because he's so good at his job that he performs procedures quickly, so he makes up the difference in income with a higher volume of patients.

I have actually lost patients because they thought I didn't charge *enough.* Can you believe it? That's because there's a certain type of patient who thinks that paying a fortune ensures them against calamities. These are often the same patients who think nothing of paying $500 for a jar of moisturizer that will barely last a month. Trying to convince them that the ingredients in the beautifully sculpted jar cost no more than a few dollars is an exercise in futility.

Myth #10: Plastic Surgery Is an Easy Fix

Cunning cosmetic surgeons know exactly how to capitalize on your fears about aging and body image, so approach any boastfulness about how easy the surgery is, how quickly you'll recover, and how the pain is "nothing to worry about" with a healthy dose of skepticism. TV shows about plastic surgery often downplay the tougher aspects of surgery, too, so it's easy to get a misguided impression that you'll waltz in for a procedure and waltz right out again, ready to go back to your life with no downtime and no downside.

No surgical procedure is an easy fix. There are risks involved. Those risks are rare, but they include blindness, permanent facial nerve injury, misshapen areas, scarring . . . and death. You also have to expect to be down for a while for recovery. There will be pain and soreness, and the body needs time to heal. It can take months for the swelling to go down before you can see the final result.

If you have realistic expectations about how you look, then you'll have real expectations about results, and you'll be happy with them.

Surgery and Smokers

From my perspective, smokers will always be poor surgical risks. Smoking constricts the body's blood vessels, decreasing blood flow to all areas, including the skin. Anyone with a decreased blood supply will be more likely to have poor wound healing, causing complications like wound breakdown, skin slough, infection, and poor scarring. This matters less with certain operations, such as breast augmentation, where the incisions are small, but for major procedures with longer incisions, such as face-lifts and tummy tucks, I will be worrying about the damage caused by constricted blood vessels. Anesthesia complications are also much higher in smokers.

For patients who are smokers, I have to be blunt. I tell them I will not operate unless they stop smoking. Obviously the best thing would be to stop for good, but if they can't and they're planning on a major procedure, such as a face-lift or tummy tuck, they can't smoke at all for two weeks before and then two weeks after the surgery.

Then I tell them about the health risks, which they do know even if they won't acknowledge them, before moving on to one of life's great motivators: money. Elective surgery is extremely costly, and smokers will always have the least optimal results, meaning they're paying more for less. If they want their face-lifts to last as long as possible, then they can't smoke. If they want their tummy tucks to be as tight as possible, then they can't smoke.

Of course, money is not the only factor. There's the time it takes to recuperate, which can be lengthy; the pain, which can be intense; the potential for scarring; and the risk of the surgery itself, which can be very real, especially for older patients or those who are overweight. Also, with the price of cigarettes today, the money saved on that carton of cigarettes can certainly be spent on other pampering necessities, like a pedicure or massage.

I try to see a patient twice before the procedure if I have any inkling that they aren't able to stop smoking. If I smell tobacco on the morning of surgery, I always cancel it. The risky potential for complications is too high.

HOW TO FIND THE BEST PLASTIC SURGEON FOR YOUR NEEDS

It's amazing how much my practice has been transformed over the years. When I was being trained in surgical techniques, the Botox that smoothes forehead wrinkles hadn't yet been created; the only injectible filler available to replace lost volume in the face was collagen; and lasers that turned out to be much more accurate than chemical peels were still years away from development. Now, of course, there's a terrific arsenal of less invasive procedures with proven results, so that you can start small instead of having a severe face-lift be your own option for sagging skin. These products, tools, and procedures are fantastic new weapons in the war on aging.

As I said before, the astounding popularity of these techniques has led to an explosion of practitioners offering them. Although it is perfectly legal for any licensed physician to perform cosmetic procedures, I'm sorry to say that many of these practitioners have little aesthetic training and can do some very real damage. The damage can be relatively small, as in a forehead treated with too much Botox, which wears off after a few months and will result in the forehead reverting to its original state. Or the damage can be catastrophic, leading to permanent disfigurement—and in the worst-case scenario: death.

Anyone considering the procedures covered in Appendixes B and C needs to do due diligence before starting any treatments. It's well worth taking a little bit of time to ask the right questions before letting just anyone help you work on improving your BQ.

Certifications and Education

One of the most important considerations in finding a plastic surgeon is to look for someone who is certified by the American Society of Plastic Surgeons (ASPS; see www.plasticsurgery.org). These surgeons have completed three to five years of a residency in general surgery, finished another two to three years of training specifically in plastic surgery, and passed extensive examinations in the specialty. This training involves the full scope of plastic surgery, not just a particular procedure or body part, and means quality treatment and appropriate follow-up care. Plus, these surgeons have met additional requirements for clinical experience and continuing education in cosmetic plastic surgery.

Sadly, any quack physician can make up a certificate claiming certification by any given "board," so it's up to you as a consumer to ascertain that the board in question is legitimate. You can check this at the Website of the American Board of Medical Specialties (ABMS; www.abms.org), the governing body of the 23 approved specialties and their board certification that exists to promote high standards of patient care.

Board-certified surgeons are also trained initially to perform reconstructive, not just cosmetic, surgery. Which means they have extensive experience with techniques performed on those who need it for medical reasons, such as burns, disfigurement due to accidents or birth defects, or reconstruction following treatment for cancer. Sure, a surgeon whose experience has nearly always been primarily with elective, aesthetic procedures may be terrifically talented, but surgeons used to dealing with the most difficult medical conditions will always have a broader depth of skill.

Many patients confuse board certification with state licensing. Individual states issue a license to practice medicine based simply upon a person having completed four years of medical school and a basic one- or two-year residency program. Board-certified plastic surgeons have gone well beyond those basic requirements.

The surgeon should also be a member of the American Society for Aesthetic Plastic Surgery (ASAPS; www.surgery.org). ASAPS surgeons and ASPS will have admitting privileges in nearby hospitals, and can only perform their procedures in accredited facilities. Be sure to ask which hospital they're affiliated with. ASAPS members must be board-certified in plastic surgery and actively engaged, in whole or in part, in all aspects of aesthetic surgery.

Word of mouth is how most patients find their surgeons, but it can backfire. If your friend gushes about the work she had done by a non–board-certified practitioner, I don't care how good she looks, you shouldn't consider risking your life with someone who hasn't had proper training and certification by the ASPS.

I can't say this strongly enough: do not go to salons, spas, or practitioners that do not have a medical license for your treatment! Some medical spas *do* employ a medical director and advertise that their procedures are monitored by that person. If the medical director is a board-certified plastic surgeon or dermatologist, this is fine, and you should be in good hands as long as the M.D. is either doing your treatment, or in the office and available during your treatment. This way, if a complication or problem arises, the doctor can be called in immediately to address it. I would be most concerned, though, if that medical director was not a plastic surgeon or dermatologist. I see "Medi-Spas" all over New York City, offering laser treatments at prices far lower than what doctors charge. But I would never let anyone put a laser within a mile of my face without knowing how much training that person has had on that specific device. Lasers aren't toys—they're dangerous, especially in unskilled hands. As I'm fond of stating: you get what you pay for!

First Consultations

Ideally, you want a surgeon who not only takes the time to talk to you and get to know you but who's also a technician with an aesthetic eye and a keen understanding of proportions and the way they relate to the face and body. During your initial consultation, the surgeon should answer all your questions in language you understand and encourage you to take notes. You should be told of all the pros, cons, and risks for any procedure you're inquiring about.

If you don't "click," then the doctor might not be the right fit for you. Sometimes a surgeon may have a bedside manner that just doesn't make you feel comfortable, and as plastic surgery involves honest conversation about expectations, you need to feel uninhibited and as relaxed as possible. Even if the surgeon has been highly recommended, you don't need to feel obligated to sign on if you have any doubts about his or her personality.

If you feel pressured in any way to consider a procedure that was not on your list, ask for detailed reasons why those suggestions are being made. Sometimes a dual procedure can reap huge rewards (eyelid lift and mini forehead lift, nose job and chin implant), but sometimes a hard sell is merely a way for the surgeon to get more business.

I always encourage patients to see at least two different surgeons for consultations prior to making a decision about whom to hire. You should hear their opinions about what work they recommend. If the facts presented to you vary considerably, you need to keep asking more questions—because someone is wrong. Or if the surgeons both give you the exact same recommendations, you can then make a choice based on personality, cost, or other factors, such as appointment availability or hospital affiliation.

If you're very anxious about your consultation, take a trusted friend or loved one with you. This person can ask questions too. I can't tell you how many times patients forget to ask questions because they're nervous—and that's totally understandable. Write your questions down beforehand and bring your list with you to the consultation.

Here are some specific questions to ask during your first consultation:

- Why do you recommend this particular procedure?
  Am I a good candidate for it?

- What are your qualifications for doing this procedure?

- How often do you update your training?

- What are the possible outcomes—good and bad? And how common are they?

- Do you have privileges to do my procedure in a hospital, and if so, which one? (This question is crucial, as hospitals will not permit unqualified surgeons to perform surgery at their institutions. And it's easy to verify this information— all you have to do is call the hospital and confirm exactly what surgical procedures your doctor is permitted to do.)

- How many procedures of this type have you performed?

- What are the risks?

- What is the pain factor going to be?

- Will I need a lot of medication?

- Do I need to have someone stay with me after surgery? For how long?

- How long is the recovery?

- When will I be able to go back to work, to the gym, or be seen in public?

- If I travel to a city away from my hometown in order to have surgery, when will I be able to leave for home? (This is another crucial question, as you need to have access to competent medical facilities should there be a post-surgical emergency.)

- Will I need to have the procedure done again, and if so, when?

- Are there other alternatives that may be less invasive or costly?

- What is your payment policy?

- What if I don't like the results?

- If a postoperative revision is needed, what, if any, are my costs?

Evaluating a Surgeon's Office or Facility

Another very important thing to consider when choosing a plastic surgeon is the facility in which they work. You should feel comfortable and in capable hands when you're in the office. If you sign on for multiple visits, you'll want to spend them in a nice environment.

So while preparing for and going on your first consultation, take a good look around and think about the office and the staff. Is the office comfortable and welcoming? How does the office staff treat you? Are they discreet? Do they return phone calls quickly? Are appointments easy to get? Do you always have a long wait to see the doctor? Are staff members willing to answer any questions?

You will also need to thoroughly vet the actual surgical suite, as many plastic surgery procedures are done on an outpatient basis in the surgeon's office. Even though the risks of these procedures are very small, your surgeon needs to be prepared for any medical emergency. Members of the American Society of Plastic Surgeons are not permitted to operate at their office facility if it is not appropriately accredited.

One of the highest standards is accreditation by the American Association for Accreditation of Ambulatory Surgery Facilities (AAAASF). These facilities must be rigorously inspected and evaluated to pass a very stringent list of codes to protect both the patient and the medical personnel, and the procedures must be performed with the most advanced instruments and monitoring devices. AAAASF accreditation also mandates monthly reporting, as well as biannual meetings with other surgeons in the area who have passed all the requirements. Each month, any complications or untoward events that occurred in the facility must be reported to the Association. Each surgeon then discusses that complication at the biannual meetings. I find these meetings to be terrifically informative and helpful—my peers and I can compare notes on our work, and share tips and techniques. This is a tremendous learning experience where colleagues discuss good and bad results, patient safety, and how to improve surgical results.

Other Considerations

While it may be fun to check out the before and after photographs in offices and on Websites, don't choose a plastic surgeon based on what you see. In the age of Photoshop and digital photography, any photo can be altered to maximize its effectiveness.

Also remember that it's smart business to check if there have been any complaints or lawsuits filed against the doctor or surgeon. You can do that by contacting your state's medical society or department of health. Bear in mind, though, that some surgeons (like obstetricians) are sued by patients who are seeking recourse for problems that may not exist or may have been caused by their own behavior (such as lying about smoking). Lawsuits have become an American way of life, unfortunately. It has become quite simple to successfully sue physicians and obtain settlements out of court because of the tort system, so you really need to look at the big picture. While some malpractice lawsuits should absolutely be filed, many others are frivolous—and they hurt everyone by pushing insurance rates up so high that many physicians are choosing not to practice high-risk procedures anymore. If a physician has been successfully sued many times, with high awards granted to the plaintiffs, you should proceed with caution.

Some lawsuits are unavoidable, however, as the practice of medicine and surgery is a science, but every patient heals differently. Unforeseen problems *can* occur and doctors can be successfully sued with minimal or no fault. (A recurring joke among my surgical colleagues is the only way to find a surgeon who has never been sued is to find one who has never performed an operation!) Bear this is mind when doing due diligence on your surgeon's reputation.

Last but not least, consider the timing of your procedure. Did you know that the most dangerous time to get a procedure done is right after a big meeting of specialists, where surgeons learn the newest techniques? If you book your operation when surgeons are eager to try what they've just learned, you might just end up being their guinea pig!

APPENDIX B

Noninvasive Procedures and Treatment Plans

OVERVIEW OF PROCEDURES

Botox

Ideal Candidate: Someone with deeply grooved glabellar (between the eyes) lines or other wrinkles/grooves on the forehead, or wrinkles around the eyes and mouth.

How It's Done: Multiple injections with a very fine syringe.

Pain Factor: Minimal; topical anesthetic cream or ice can be used.

Recuperation/Downtime: None. There may be slight bruising, which is easily covered with makeup.

How Bad You'll Really Look: Like nothing happened, as it takes hours to start to work, so you can go back to work afterward.

What Could Go Wrong: There could be a temporary upper eyelid droop.

When You'll See Results: Usually within 1–14 days.

How Long It Lasts: Three to six months.

Inside Scoop: Botox is a type A toxin, a highly purified protein produced by the *Clostridium botulinum* bacterium. It works by blocking the nerve impulses that signal muscles to move. No movement of the muscles under the skin means no wrinkling of the skin above them. But it's not that simple; injecting Botox should still be thought of as an art, because you need to take the arch of the brows, the shape of the forehead, a patient's age, and especially the skin's elasticity into consideration.

In other words, having a "Botox party," where someone whose credentials are not particularly stellar goes around injecting people, is asking for trouble! Especially if the lines around the mouth are being treated—a quack might affect your ability to eat or swallow.

Dermabrasion and Microdermabrasion

Before there were effective lasers, anyone needing serious exfoliation would have considered dermabrasion. Because it literally scrapes off several layers of skin, it's often used to lighten or remove some scars. Obviously, you should consider dermabrasion only when you need a heavy-duty treatment for wrinkles, aging, and pigmentation problems.

Microdermabrasion, on the other hand, uses a different tool, and removes only the very topmost layer of skin with a fine spray of aluminum oxide crystals. It's such a gentle procedure that most people can have a treatment at lunchtime and then go right back to work, with only a little makeup to cover up potential redness.

Ideal Candidate: Dermabrasion is for patients with deep wrinkles, acne scars, or some facial scars. It must be noted, however, that regular dermabrasion is used less frequently today because of the advancement and refinement of lasers, which treat the same conditions—and usually with more precision. Still, dermabrasion can be effective, especially when combined with a chemical peel.

Microdermabrasion works well for those with fine wrinkles, or who wish to have the ultimate facial, especially when combined with a mild chemical peel.

How It's Done: Dermabrasion utilizes a handheld device with a rough brush or a diamond burr, and mechanically removes layers of skin. For microdermabrasion, aluminum oxide crystals are used like a mini sandblaster.

Pain Factor: Dermabrasion does require mild postoperative pain management with analgesics, but microdermabrasion, with or without a mild chemical peel, is painless and the patient may return to work or go out to dinner that evening.

Recuperation/Downtime: Dermabrasion requires two to seven days to heal and allow coverage with makeup. Microdermabrasion has no downtime at all.

How Bad You'll Really Look: With dermabrasion, pretty bad for a few days, with scabs and redness.

What Could Go Wrong: There is a possibility of infection and, rarely, worse scarring.

When You'll See Results: For dermabrasion, two to six weeks. Microdermabrasion has immediate results. Dermabrasion can be repeated four to six months later, or at a much later date. Microdermabrasion can and should be done three or four times a year, or whenever you normally would get a facial as an alternative.

How Long It Lasts: Lifetime, with dermabrasion. Microdermabrasion is more of a skin maintenance regimen.

Inside Scoop: Because dermabrasion involves rough scraping, you should never consider this procedure unless it is done by skilled, experienced hands. Otherwise you could be badly scarred, with skin that's blotchy and uneven.

But because dermabrasion goes deep, the results can be remarkable. It's also highly effective for those with acne scarring. But as I've said, precision laser technology has placed both these options further back on our skin-care shelf.

As with untrained or supervised laser wielders, micro-dermabrasion is often available at nail salons or spas and performed by nonmedical personnel without supervision of a doctor. This is dangerous, in my opinion, and asking for trouble. Stick to a practitioner with a medical license and expertise. You only have one face!

Fillers—Injectible

Ideal Candidate: Someone who's lost volume in her face. As we age, fat in the face falls and dissipates, which means that it no longer fills out the face, leading to more wrinkling.

How It's Done: The filler material hyaluronic acid (Restylane or Juvederm) is injected into the face. Fat can also be harvested via liposuction from other parts of your body and then injected.

Pain Factor: Minimal; topical numbing cream can be used.

Recuperation/Downtime: One to two days.

How Bad You'll Really Look: A bit swollen and bruised for a few days.

What Could Go Wrong: Undercorrection, overcorrection, uneven correction, or, rarely, clumping of the filler.

When You'll See Results: Immediately.

How Long It Lasts: Hyaluronic acid last three to six months. Fat transfer varies; some of the fat will remain while the rest of it may be absorbed by the body, requiring one to two more procedures for a longer-lasting result.

Inside Scoop: The secret to good results with fillers is to still look like yourself—only a little bit better. But as with Botox, too much filler leads to unnaturally puffy and smooth faces and cheeks. Women of a certain age are certainly not expected to be entirely wrinkle-free—and if they are, their BQ goes way down as they just don't look natural. They look rather *stuffed!* So as with an aesthetic procedure, a light touch is much better for a high BQ than a heavy hand. You can always add more.

Lasers and Other Light Sources

Ideal Candidate: Someone with moderate wrinkles, sun damage, uneven skin tone, pigmentation spots, and/or widened pores.

How It's Done: The laser burns away the outer layers of the face, removing damaged skin and allowing fresh, new skin to take its place.

Pain Factor: Moderate; easily controlled by pain medication.

Recuperation/Downtime: Three to seven days, depending upon the power settings used. Deeper, more sun-damaged skin requires higher power settings and a longer recovery. The fractional CO_2 laser requires three to five days. Laser technology keeps improving, and better results and shorter downtimes will result.

How Bad You'll Really Look: With lower laser settings, it'll look like a sunburn; higher settings make your skin look like burnt toast for one to two days.

What Could Go Wrong: Rarely, poor healing with scarring. The laser might also cause hyperpigmentation or hypopigmentation, which is usually temporary.

When You'll See Results: After the dead skin peels away, usually within two to four weeks.

How Long It Lasts: One to three years.

Inside Scoop: Talk about confusing. There are so many new lasers out there that I always tell my patients that I don't buy lasers—I rent them. That's because lasers keep improving, so it's easier to use the latest device when I don't have the financial obligation of buying it.

My laser of choice right now is the fractional CO2, as the ablative part (what causes the heat) is not as aggressive as in other lasers but with the same effective penetration down into damaged skin, so you'll look sunburned but not deep-fried after treatment.

I'm not a fan of other light treatments, such as IPL (Intense Pulsed Light) or Fraxel, because some patients have decent results while others get no improvement. So if a device is inconsistent, I'll always hesitate to use it on my patients. They deserve to know that they'll get proven results.

Peels

How It's Done: Various types of acid or chemicals essentially burn away outer skin layers, allowing fresh new skin to replace them.

Pain Factor: Moderate; easily controlled by pain medication.

Recuperation/Downtime: Three to five days.

How Bad You'll Really Look: Like burnt toast for one to three days, then dead skin peels away, revealing pink healthy skin; easily covered by makeup.

What Could Go Wrong: Rarely, poor healing with scarring and/or hyperpigmentation; hypopigmentation is usually temporary.

When You'll See Results: After the dead skin peels away, usually within two to four weeks.

How Long It Lasts: Two to five years.

Inside Scoop: As chemical peels usually have the same downtime and after-effects as lasers—but are slightly less effective—I prefer to use lasers, since they offer more control regarding the depth of skin treated (which is impossible to do with chemical peels). But for the right candidates, mild chemical peels have proven results and are still an excellent choice.

FACE, HEAD, AND NECK

Cheeks—Lack Definition

Procedure: Fillers or fat transfer.

Inside Scoop: I prefer to do a fat transfer rather than use fillers to improve cheeks, but you may need more than one procedure. Fillers can clump together in an unnatural fashion, so the end result is cheeks that are noticeably too plump, creating a chipmunk look. Fat transfer provides a more natural improvement.

Chin—Too Prominent

Procedure: Fillers that improve the contours of the cheeks might be able to make a prominent chin less noticeable, but surgery is usually the only option. See Appendix C.

Chin—Too Weak

Procedure: Fillers or fat transfer can provide modest improvement.

Inside Scoop: Filling up a weak chin is tricky and a skillful hand is a must. Otherwise, any inappropriate placement of the fillers or fat can look phony and ridiculous.

Ears—Sticking Out

Procedure: If a good haircut isn't enough to hide your ears, surgery is your only option. See Appendix C.

Eyes—Bags/Circles Under Lower Lid

Procedure: Retin A for mild cases; laser resurfacing, or chemical peel for darker circles.

Inside Scoop: Retin A is one of the few FDA-approved treatments for fine lines and wrinkles, and since it's noninvasive, inexpensive, and absolutely works, it's worth trying on your eye bags. Be sure to use sunscreen religiously, as any use of Retin A makes the delicate skin in the area far more susceptible to sun damage. Retin A can also cause significant irritation for those with sensitive skin, which may require use every other day or every third day and a more diluted solution. I recommend using Retin A in the evening, allowing it to work while you're asleep, and then always applying a super-hydrating moisturizer in the morning.

Eyes—Crepey and/or Excess Skin on Upper Lid

Procedure: Laser resurfacing or chemical peel—judiciously.

Inside Scoop: Once the skin texture changes or elasticity is gone, it's gone for good, so excess eyelid skin is very difficult to treat without surgery. Lasers or peels can be used in this region, but only by a very experienced physician. This is one area where surgery might actually be the safer option because the upper eyelid skin is the thinnest on the body, and is easily damaged. See Appendix C.

Face—Age Spots

Procedure: Lasers and chemical peels.

Inside Scoop: Lasers and/or chemical peels are used to treat, remove, and even out pigmentation issues, especially dark spots and irregularities caused by long-term sun exposure. Each patient's skin type dictates which procedure will be most helpful. Again, it is vital to seek treatment from a board-certified dermatologist or plastic surgeon when dealing with hyperpigmentation (brown spots) or hypopigmentation (white spots). The wrong treatment can worsen the problem, and can be difficult to correct.

Face—Deep Grooves (Nasolabial Fold)

Procedure: Moderate grooves can be treated with fillers or fat transfer.

Inside Scoop: If the folds are not too bad, and the rest of the face still in decent shape, go for fillers first—as long as you have realistic expectations, as the grooves can only be softened, not completely removed. Nor do you want to completely remove these grooves, as they're caused by the muscles that allow us to smile!

But if you do need a lot of syringes, the cost can quickly add up and be nearly as high as a face-lift (if not higher). If so, and if you're in good health, surgery is by far a more long-lasting and cost-effective treatment. See Appendix C.

Face—Fine Wrinkles

Procedure: Microdermabrasion, light chemical or acid peels, or mild lasers.

Inside Scoop: If you're not seeing results with OTC creams and serums, microdermabrasion is an effective treatment with little if any side effects (save for some redness), and can be repeated every four to six weeks.

Don't get talked into injectible fillers for fine wrinkles if you don't really need them! Fillers are expensive, and they work when wrinkles are more pronounced.

Face—Moderate to Severe Wrinkles

Procedure: Fractional CO2 laser resurfacing; filler.

Inside Scoop: Laser resurfacing is an effective, less-invasive procedure than a face-lift. It really does remove fine lines and damaged skin, closes wide pores, and modestly tightens the face, improving the deeper wrinkles, too.

Injectible fillers can smooth out wrinkles, too, as when they replace lost volume, they plump up the skin's appearance. Combining laser resurfacing with fillers can provide excellent improvement for the right candidate, avoiding the need for a face-lift.

Face—Sagging/Wrinkles/Jowls

Procedure: Fillers or fat transfer (for moderate sagging only).

Inside Scoop: Fillers replace lost volume in the face, but they can't fix droopy folds or jowls, or serious sagging. So if new patients are either overdone or need surgical lifting, I tell them that using fillers at this point is like spitting in the ocean. In fact, I won't do the injections—unless the patient is adamant that she doesn't want a face-lift and is willing to spend the tens of thousands of dollars it will cost, and will commit to redoing her whole face every six months or so.

Often, more really is less; a face-lift might be surgery, but once it's done, it'll last for many years (not months).

Forehead—Sagging

Procedure: Botox or fillers.

Inside Scoop: Sometimes Botox placed in the appropriate location can lift a sagging forehead modestly but nicely. Fillers only fill in the wrinkles of the forehead, helping to mask the sagging aspect.

Forehead—Too High/Prominent

Procedure: Aside from getting a good haircut with bangs, you'll need surgery to treat this condition. See Appendix C.

Forehead—Wrinkles/Frown Lines

Procedure: Botox.

Inside Scoop: It's hard to believe that only a few short years ago, botulism was something you didn't want to get if you valued your stomach (and your life). Now, of course, Botox is the most common procedure performed by plastic surgeons. It's such a big business that countless Hollywood foreheads have been smoothed so seamlessly that casting directors are going bonkers trying to find actresses over 30 who can still frown and furrow their brows.

Be very judicious with Botox, as it's way too easy to get carried away, and erase all signs of character in your face! It's very easy to lower your BQ when your ultra-smooth forehead doesn't match the rest of your face or body.

Hair—Loss

Procedure: If you don't respond well to Rogaine or other hair regrowth creams, the only option is surgery. See Appendix C.

Lips—Too Thin

Procedure: Fillers such as hyaluronic acid, collagen, or fat transfer.

Inside Scoop: Conservative augmentation with a very small amount of filler can look completely natural, especially as lips tend to get thinner as we age. But overplumping will be sure to get you the kind of attention you'd rather not have, particularly if you end up looking like Daffy Duck—what some popular magazines and newspapers tabloids have come to call "trout pout."

Older versions of collagen are derived from cows, so you'll need allergy testing prior to use; newer collagen products no longer require testing. And as lips become swollen after the injections, you'll look more pouty for a day or so. Bear this in mind when scheduling your appointment.

Neck—Prominent Muscle (Platysmal Bands)

Procedure: Botox injections, if you do not have excess skin and/or fat in the neck.

Inside Scoop: As the platysmal bands can become very prominent as we age, Botox can work wonders, sparing you the need for surgery.

Neck—Sagging/Jowly

Procedure: Fillers provide improvement in patients with very minor sagging.

Inside Scoop: For moderate to serious sagging, this is one location where surgery really is the only option. See Appendix C.

Nose—Botched Nose Job

Procedure: Surgery is the only option. See Appendix C.

Nose—Overly Large/Crooked

Procedure: Some dermatologists or surgeons use a small injection of Botox at the base of the nose to lift up the tip, but I am not a fan of this procedure as it doesn't always work. Often, only the doctor and the patient notice improvement, if any. Otherwise, surgery is your only option. See Appendix C.

BODY

If you've tried all the suggestions in Chapter 7 for breasts, buttocks, or excess skin, and still aren't satisfied, you might want to move on to surgical options described in Appendix C. The only part of the body that can be treated with a noninvasive procedure is the hands.

Hands—Crepey/Thin/Mottled Skin

Procedure: Fillers, such as Restylane, plump up the loss of underlying fat. For age spots, lasers or chemical peels are the best option.

Inside Scoop: Be aware that the amount of filler you might need to plump up your hands could cost a small fortune!

Plastic Surgery Procedures and Treatment Plans

FACE, HEAD, AND NECK

Cheeks—Lack Definition

Ideal Candidate: Person with some definition of cheek region, otherwise the results can be too extreme or look obviously fake; nonsmoker.

Procedure: Cheek implants.

How It's Done: Artificial implants placed over cheekbones to increase definition.

Pain Factor: Moderate; easily controlled by pain medication.

Recuperation/Downtime: You'll be very swollen for one to two weeks.

How Bad You'll Really Look: You could be bruised, swollen, and scary-looking for three to five days.

What Could Go Wrong: Infection; implants can become displaced, or they can just look terrible, requiring removal.

When You'll See Results: Immediately.

How Long It Lasts: Lifetime.

Inside Scoop: Cheek implants, when done properly, can make a big difference in your appearance. Always err on the side of smaller rather than larger; if they're too big they'll look ridiculously fake. However, if they move or become dislodged, they must be surgically removed.

Chin—Too Prominent

Ideal Candidate: One with minor deformity.

Procedure: Burr down chin bone.

How It's Done: Power burr reduces bone mass in chin region.

Pain Factor: High; strong pain medication is a must.

Recuperation/Downtime: One to two weeks, bruising and swelling.

How Bad You'll Really Look: Like a power tool was taken to your chin—because it was!

What Could Go Wrong: Removal of too much of bone.

When You'll See Result: Two to four weeks after the swelling goes down.

How Long It Lasts: Lifetime.

Inside Scoop: This is not a common procedure. Look at it this way: a prominent chin hasn't hurt Jay Leno's career!

Chin—Too Weak

Ideal Candidate: One with moderate deformity.

Procedure: Chin implant.

How It's Done: Implant placed over jawbone in chin region.

Pain Factor: Moderate; easily controlled with pain medication.

Recuperation/Downtime: One week.

How Bad You'll Really Look: Swollen and bruised for a couple of days.

What Could Go Wrong: Infection; implant displacement requiring removal.

When You'll See Results: One to two weeks after the swelling goes down.

How Long It Lasts: Lifetime.

Inside Scoop: This is an excellent procedure for patients with modestly weak chins. It's often performed in conjunction with a rhinoplasty for a patient with a prominent nose. The combination of decreasing the size of the nose while increasing the chin region provides a more natural correction. Patients with severely weak chins require a more invasive procedure, which includes fracturing and advancing the jawbone forward to correct the deformity.

Ears—Sticking Out

Ideal Candidate: One with mild or severe deformities.

Procedure: Otoplasty—pin ears back.

How It's Done: Some ear cartilage may or may not need to be removed and permanent sutures placed to hold ear in corrected position. Scar is hidden behind each ear.

Pain Factor: Modest; easily controlled by pain medication.

Recuperation/Downtime: Three to five days.

How Bad You'll Really Look: Your ears may be bruised and swollen for three to five days.

What Could Go Wrong: Under- or overcorrection, both of which can easily be fixed; hematoma (blood under the skin).

When You'll See Results: Immediately.

How Long It Lasts: Lifetime.

Inside Scoop: Luckily, this is an excellent procedure with high levels of patient satisfaction. It's often and easily performed on children who are being teased or bullied at a young age by their peers. Adults who have lived a life of covering their ears with their hair are thrilled to celebrate their ability to cut their hair or pull it back in a ponytail after this operation.

Eyes—Bags/Circles Under Lower Lid

Ideal Candidate: Lower eyelid blepharoplasty, with excess skin resection.

Procedure: Excess fat is removed or pushed back through an incision under the eyelid or just inside the eye (leaving no scar).

How It's Done: Excess fat is removed or pushed back in, and excess skin may or may not need to be cut away.

Pain Factor: Modest; easily controlled by pain medication.

Recuperation/Downtime: One week.

How Bad You'll Really Look: Swollen and bruised for five to seven days.

What Could Go Wrong: Blindness (which is incredibly rare); over-resection of the skin, causing the lower lid to pull down, preventing closure of eye, dry eyes, and deformity.

When You'll See Results: As soon as the swelling goes down.

How Long It Lasts: Usually, a lifetime; sometimes a small amount of excess skin may need to be removed in 10–20 years.

Inside Scoop: A model once came to me when she was just starting out. She was 19 and incredibly striking, but she had exceptionally thin and delicate skin under her eyes and wanted the "bags" removed. After I examined her, I told her that she didn't have "bags," but that her skin was so thin under her eyes that what she thought was fat was actually normal muscle, and I didn't think it should be touched. And then I urged her to wait six months, and if she found that photographers were complaining that her muscle was causing shadows, to come back and I'd reconsider. Well, I was so glad she listened to me, because I saw her on a magazine cover three months later, her gorgeous eyes untouched. I lost a patient, but felt pretty darn good!

Eyes—Crepey Skin on Upper Lid

Ideal Candidate: Thin, overly loose crepey skin on the upper eyelids.

Procedure: Upper eyelid blepharoplasty, where excess skin is removed.

How It's Done: Excess upper eyelid skin is cut away.

Pain Factor: Moderate; easily controlled by pain medication.

Recuperation/Downtime: Five to seven days.

How Bad You'll Really Look: Swollen and bruised for five to seven days.

What Could Go Wrong: Blindness (which is incredibly rare); too much skin removed, so that the upper eyelid can no longer pull down, leaving you unable to close your eyes entirely, which can then cause chronic dry eyes and a deformity.

When You'll See Results: As soon as the swelling goes down.

How Long It Lasts: Usually a lifetime; sometimes a small amount of excess skin may need to be removed in 10–20 years.

Inside Scoop: This is a very popular procedure, as the scar, hidden in the fold of the upper eyelid, fades nicely with time and is easily covered with makeup as early as one week after the surgery. Patients look rested and rejuvenated, without seeming to have had any major work done. I've found that men in executive positions, concerned that they look sleepy or inattentive during afternoon meetings, often love this the "bleph," as it is called.

I do a lot of mini brow lifts when I do eyelids, too, since the eyebrows naturally descend as you age, contributing to the excess skin on the eyelids. There is something called a lower frontal bone on the lower forehead where your eyebrows used to sit when you were younger. I always tell my patients that if I just do the eyelids, I can take out only a little skin and they'll still look tired, but if I take out too much skin without lifting the brows they're going to look ridiculous; their eyebrows will be resting in a very low position. Most of my patients don't believe me when I tell them about this— they think I'm trying to tack on an extra procedure. I'm talking about only gently lifting, which will make a huge difference. When I hold up a mirror and slightly lift their eyebrows, it lifts some of the redundant skin away from the eyelids, and softens their stern appearance, driving home my point.

Face—Age Spots

Procedure: The only time surgery is needed for pigmentation problems is when a mole or spot turns cancerous. Otherwise, lasers or peels are your best bet. See Appendix B.

Face—Deep Grooves (Nasolabial Fold)

Ideal Candidate: One with realistic expectations.

Procedure: Severe grooves require a face-lift (see Face—Sagging/ Wrinkles/Jowls).

Face—Fine Wrinkles

Procedure: Usually, a face-lift is overkill if there are only fine wrinkles on a face. Still, a face-lift can be extremely effective if fine lines and wrinkles are present all over the face. Each particular case needs to be evaluated (see Face—Sagging/Wrinkles/Jowls).

Face—Moderate to Severe Wrinkles

Procedure: Your best bet is a face-lift. See Face—Sagging/Wrinkles/ Jowls.

Face—Sagging/Wrinkles/Jowls

Ideal Candidate: One with realistic expectations, who understands which areas can be treated and how she'll be improved; nonsmoker.

Procedure: Face-lift.

How It's Done: Various surgical techniques, depending upon severity of problem.

Pain Factor: Moderate; easily controlled by pain medication.

Recuperation/Downtime: One to two weeks.

How Bad You'll Really Look: Like you went a few rounds with the champ. Actually, it depends on the procedure, as newer techniques are less invasive with shorter scars.

What Could Go Wrong: Facial nerve injury, hematoma, poor scarring, the super-fake, overstretched, wind tunnel look!

When You'll See Results: Two to four weeks after the swelling goes down.

How Long It Last: Depending on the procedure, the patient's age and quality of skin, usually 3–15 years.

Inside Scoop: A great tip if you're considering a face-lift is to lie down on your back and hold a mirror up. What this does is reposition the structure in your face, since gravity is no longer a factor when you're lying down. Voila—your face is back to what it used to be. And, no, it's not going to be pulled to the side and back, which gives you that dreaded and obviously overstretched profile.

Forehead—Sagging

Ideal Candidate: Someone who's tired of Botox's temporary-only results, or with a chronically angry or tired look; nonsmoker.

Procedure: Mini brow lift, endoscopic brow lift, open brow lift.

How It's Done: Through small incisions in hair-bearing scalp, or long incision in same region.

Pain Factor: Modest; easily controlled by pain medication.

Recuperation/Downtime: One to two weeks.

How Bad You'll Really Look: Moderate swelling and bruising.

What Could Go Wrong: Poor scarring causing alopecia (hair loss, which is easily fixed); or overcorrection, creating that constant surprised look.

When You'll See Results: Two to four weeks after the swelling goes down.

How Long It Lasts: Five to ten years.

Inside Scoop: When done well, and in a conservative fashion, a regular or mini brow lift is an excellent adjunct to a face-lift or eye tuck.

Forehead—Too High/Prominent

Ideal Candidate: Nonsmoker.

Procedure: Open brow lift with the incision placed at anterior (front) hairline, allowing excess skin to be removed from the forehead, lowering the scalp and anterior headline, decreasing forehead prominence.

How It's Done: This requires an incision at the hairline, so only excess forehead skin is removed, decreasing prominence.

Pain Factor: Moderate; easily controlled by pain medication.

Recuperation/Downtime: One week.

How Bad You'll Really Look: Swollen and bruised.

What Could Go Wrong: Hematoma, prominent scar showing at the hairline.

When You'll See Results: Two to four weeks after the swelling goes down.

How Long It Lasts: Lifetime.

Inside Scoop: It's an effective procedure, but one that requires expert technique to hide the scar.

Forehead—Wrinkles

Procedure: Discuss your options for a brow lift with your plastic surgeon. Otherwise, Botox is an excellent option. See Chapter 7.

Hair—Loss

Ideal Candidate: Someone with moderate hair loss, which is stable.

Procedure: Hair transplant.

How It's Done: Strips of hair are taken from the posterior portion of scalp, then cut up into small plugs with one to three hairs in each plug and placed in the region of the scalp lacking hair.

Pain Factor: Minimal.

Recuperation/Downtime: One to two weeks; must wear hat.

How Bad You'll Really Look: A hat is required for at least one week.

What Could Go Wrong: The grafts won't take, or if the plugs are too large, the result can be a cobblestone and obviously fake appearance. The scars can be noticeable.

When You'll See Results: Three to six months.

How Long It Lasts: Lifetime.

Inside Scoop: A newer technique, taking microplugs of one or two hairs per plug, has revolutionized this procedure, creating a very natural result.

Lips—Too Thin

Procedure: I'd advise you to steer clear of surgical correction to lift the upper lip and make it look more plump. These procedures leave scars, which may be prominent, and if you're unhappy with the result, undoing any lip surgery will leave even more unsightly scars.

Fillers are far more effective and look more natural when performed correctly. And fillers wear off, so if you're unhappy with the results you don't have to live with them forever!

Neck—Prominent Muscle (Platysmal Bands)

Ideal Candidate: Someone with prominent muscle bands in the neck; nonsmoker.

Procedure: If you have excess skin and/or fat in the neck, a mini face/neck lift.

How It's Done: In some cases the prominent bands can be corrected through an incision just under the chin if there is minimal redundant skin; otherwise the incision in front of the ear must be used.

Pain Factor: Moderate; easily controlled by pain medication.

Recuperation/Downtime: Five to ten days.

How Bad You'll Really Look: Bruised and swollen.

What Could Go Wrong: Early recurrence of prominent bands, hematoma.

When You'll See Results: Two to four weeks after the swelling goes down.

How Long It Lasts: Three to eight years.

Inside Scoop: Try Botox first. You know my motto by now: the less invasive, the better.

Neck—Sagging/Jowls

Ideal Candidate: Redundant skin and excess fat in the neck region with muscle bands protruding (platysmal banding); nonsmoker.

Procedure: Mini face/neck lift.

How It's Done: A small incision is made in front of the ear, the neck is tightened and excess skin trimmed.

Pain Factor: Moderate; easily controlled by pain medication.

Recuperation/Downtime: Five to ten days.

How Bad You'll Really Look: Swollen and bruised.

What Could Go Wrong: Hematoma, facial nerve injury (though this is rare).

When You'll See Results: Two to four weeks after the swelling goes down.

How Long It Lasts: Six to ten years.

Inside Scoop: Necks are usually neglected, so they're often the first area to show distinct signs of aging. A correction is an excellent way to put sand back in the hourglass!

Nose—Botched Nose Job

Ideal Candidate: Realistic expectations; nonsmoker.

Procedure: Open rhinoplasty.

How It's Done: A small incision is made on the columella (the area of nose just above the lip) allowing greater access to all areas of the nose. Corrections can include cartilage grafts and nasal tip refinement, leaving a small scar that becomes nearly imperceptible in six months to a year.

Pain Factor: Moderate; easily controlled by pain medication.

Recuperation/Downtime: One to two weeks. No exercise for four to six weeks.

How Bad You'll Really Look: As swollen and bruised as with your first nose job.

What Could Go Wrong: Inadequate improvement of problems or even worsening.

When You'll See Results: As with a regular rhinoplasty, six weeks to 12 months for the final result.

How Long It Lasts: Lifetime.

Inside Scoop: One of the weirdest things I've ever seen was during a training course on noses, in Dallas, where we practiced procedures on cadavers. We met in an enormous room in a medical school, with tables neatly lined up in a row—and with a severed head on each of them. It was like a horror movie, only with plastic surgeons and surgical residents gowned up, scalpels in hand. See, bodies are very hard to come by for medical schools now, so everything is used.

I'm very grateful I had this hands-on training, because if you mess up a nose the first time, you've got a problem. I did my first few live noses under the direct supervision of a surgeon much more senior than myself, who walked me through each and every step until I had the confidence and skill to do it on my own. Take a look at all the botched nose jobs out there and you'll understand how tricky the procedure is. You've always got to be careful and meticulous.

Take the actress Jennifer Grey, the star of *Dirty Dancing*. She was absolutely adorable in that film, with a large nose that gave her a distinctive panache. Well, she decided to have a nose job several years later, and as soon as she saw the results she admitted (in many interviews over the years) that she'd made a terrible mistake. Her new nose was gorgeous. The surgery hadn't been botched at all, and she looked lovely. But she'd lost that essential element that had made her so unique, and there was no way to undo the damage. Even though she was more classically beautiful with her new nose, her BQ changed because she looked like a thousand other actresses—not her previous, unique self.

Nose—Overly Large/Crooked

Ideal Candidate: Large crooked nose that is too large or misshapen for the patient's face.

Procedure: Rhinoplasty, open or closed; nonsmoker.

How It's Done: Excess bone and cartilage is trimmed and sculpted to reduce the size, improve the shape, and improve nasal breathing if nasal septum is involved. Sometimes the nasal bone must be broken to achieve good results.

Pain Factor: Moderate, easily controlled by pain medication.

Recuperation/Downtime: Five to seven days. No exercise two to four weeks.

How Bad You'll Really Look: Swollen and bruised, especially under the eyes.

What Could Go Wrong: Overachievement or underachievement of goals, resulting in a nose that does not fit the face; worsening of nasal breathing problems and bleeding early in recovery period.

When You'll See Results: You'll see noticeable results about six weeks after the procedure, as it takes a long time for the swelling to go down. You'll see final results in 6–12 months.

How Long It Lasts: The result, good or bad, lasts a lifetime, so choose your surgeon well!

Inside Scoop: This is one of the few operations that requires the plastic surgeon to possess the skills of a sculptor. The surgeon must mold bone, cartilage, and skin in a creative fashion for optimal results. The best chance for a great result is a "virgin nose," secondary rhinoplasties are much more complicated.

BODY

Breasts—Cancer/Reconstruction

Ideal Candidate: A patient who's lost breast(s) from breast cancer; nonsmoker. Reconstruction can be performed at the time of mastectomy or at a later date.

Procedure: These include transfer of tissue from the tummy to the chest, allowing for a tummy tuck at the same time; transfer of tissue from the back, or placement of a tissue expander (balloon) followed by placement of permanent implant, usually silicone.

How It's Done: Usually in the hospital or surgery center.

Pain Factor: Moderate to significant, depending on the procedure; well controlled by pain medication.

Recuperation/Downtime: Two to six weeks, depending on the procedure.

How Bad You'll Really Look: It depends upon the procedure. Some allow the patient to wake up with a breast mound immediately after the mastectomy; when tissue expanders are used, you'll have to go back for several weeks to have them expanded, but in a very short while breast mounds appear, easing the loss of the breast.

What Could Go Wrong: Flap loss, infection, rejection of tissue expander.

When You'll See Results: It depends on the procedure: immediately with the flap, and three to six months with the tissue expander.

How Long It Lasts: Flap surgery (autologous tissue) lasts a lifetime. Tissue expander followed by permanent implant will require an exchange of the implant in 10–15 years.

Inside Scoop: I can do a phenomenal face-lift yet still have the patient come to me a few months later and say, "Well, I'm really not happy about this one wrinkle. You couldn't get rid of this one wrinkle?" Yet with my breast reconstruction patients it's a completely different mind-set. I always want to do a little more tweaking to make reconstructed breasts look even better and I often hear, "Are you kidding? You don't need to touch them—they're perfect!"

You should also be aware that federal law now *requires* insurance companies to pay for breast reconstruction after mastectomy for cancer, as well as surgery on the opposite breast to provide symmetry. Breast reconstruction after cancer is considered an integral part of breast cancer treatment.

Breasts—Sagging

Ideal Candidate: Women with shapeless, sagging breasts, sometimes below the inframammary fold and who have also lost volume, often after childbirth and/or breastfeeding; nonsmoker.

Procedure: Mastopexy, or breast lift.

How It's Done: Various procedures causing various scar formations, depending on the shape and sag of the breasts.

Pain Factor: Moderate to minimal for 24–48 hours, easily controlled with pain medication.

Recuperation/Downtime: Five to seven days from work. No exercise for one to two weeks.

How Bad You'll Really Look: Immediate improvement, although breasts may appear too high initially but will settle within six weeks.

When You'll See Results: Immediately, and this will improve greatly over time as the swelling gradually goes down.

What Could Go Wrong: Infection, hematoma, decreased sensation or loss of sensation to nipples—all these complications are rare but poor scarring can be an issue.

How Long It Lasts: That depends on the procedure and the patient's skin type. Also weight gain, weight loss, or pregnancy have a strong effect on longevity, but it's usually 5–15 years.

Inside Scoop: Patient satisfaction level is high, especially for moms who get their "pre-baby boobs" back. A note of caution: many patients request a breast lift (mastopexy) along with breast augmentation, called augmentation mastopexy. The combination is a much more complicated procedure, requiring experience and expertise.

Severely sagging breasts—sort of shaped like sausages or the Peanuts' character Snoopy's nose, are called constricted breasts. They're usually cause for intense embarrassment. One of the toughest operations I ever did was on a woman with incredibly constricted breasts. It was one of the most difficult operations I ever performed, and I was telling this to the patient's sister afterward, while the patient was in the recovery room. "You'll know how complicated this was once you see the result," I explained.

"No, I won't," the sister replied. That's how inhibited the patient had been—no one, not even a beloved sister—had ever seen her breasts.

Happily, the patient was ecstatic with her new breast shape, and helping her was one of the most satisfying experiences of my career.

Breasts—Too Large

Ideal Candidate: A woman with extremely large breasts creating physical deformities, backache, headaches, ridging of the shoulders from brassiere straps, chronic skin conditions; nonsmoker.

Procedure: Breast reduction.

How It's Done: Various techniques involving various scar locations, depending on the size and shape of the breasts.

Pain Factor: Moderate, lasting 24–48 hours; easily controlled with pain medication.

Recuperation/Downtime: Away from work one week. No exercise for two to four weeks.

How Bad You'll Really Look: Improvement is immediate, although there will be some swelling for one to two weeks after surgery.

What Could Go Wrong: Infection, hematoma, decreased nipple sensation, poor scarring, and, very rarely, nipple loss. You should still be able to breastfeed.

When You'll See Results: Immediately, with continued improvement as scars fade over time.

How Long It Lasts: Results are permanent without excessive weight gain or loss or pregnancy. With age, they may sag.

Inside Scoop: As with severe sagging, this operation has one of the highest levels of postoperative satisfaction. Patients describe their relief as, literally, that a giant "weight has been lifted from their shoulders." Even better, trading scars for normal-sized and attractively shaped breasts is easily (and gratefully) accepted by most patients.

Breasts—Too Small

Ideal Candidate: Woman with small breasts and realistic expectations.

Procedure: Breast augmentation with silicone or saline implants.

How It's Done: Implants can be placed above or below the muscle through incisions in the breast crease, around the areola, or the armpit.

Pain Factor: Under the muscle will be more painful than over the muscle, but discomfort lasts 24–48 hours; easily controlled with pain medication.

Recuperation/Downtime: Away from work five to seven days. No exercise for one to four weeks.

How Bad You'll Really Look: Initially, you'll look and feel tight, which lasts for about one to two weeks. The breasts will feel like they are yours after six months.

What Could Go Wrong: Bleeding, asymmetry, decreased nipple sensation, infection requiring removal of the implants—all these complications are rare.

When You'll See Results: Immediately, but for women with small breasts, the skin and muscle need to stretch, so the shape will improve over three to six months. My patients tell me that they feel like "their own breasts again" after six months.

How Long It Lasts: I always tell patients that if they decide to get implants, they are signing up for at least one more operation. Breast implants are *not* permanent and need to be changed every 10–12 years. I equate this to changing a tire—with normal wear and tear, there's just a small cut and a quick replacement.

Extreme weight loss, weight gain, or pregnancy will affect the breast shape, possibly requiring revision.

Inside Scoop: This operation can have a high level of satisfaction when the patient has realistic expectations, and she's doing the operation for the right person: *herself!* I tell my patients that if they want this procedure and are willing to have their bodies cut solely to please their husband or boyfriend, they're making a mistake.

Be very wary of a surgeon who encourages you to go from an A cup to a large D cup (or bigger). The best results are the most natural results, which tends to mean small changes—from an A to a B, or a B to a C. I think the best results come from when your body is properly proportioned, unless you are a professional stripper.

I often ask my patients to bring in photos of breasts they like, as most women don't know what a true A, B, C, or larger cup size really looks like. I also have actual cups so patients can put one in their current-sized bras to see what they look like with a larger size.

The real art is taking someone unhappy with a certain part of her body and then giving her confidence about her new appearance. I love it when a woman who initially comes in for a consultation is covered up or conservatively dressed—and then after the breast augmentation there's a complete metamorphosis!

Buttocks—Too Large

Ideal Candidate: A patient with realistic expectations, and who was unable to accomplish her goals with diet, vigorous exercise, and weight training.

Procedure: Liposuction. See Excess Skin—Fat Deposits in Specific Areas.

Inside Scoop: Liposuction in the buttocks can be a double-edged sword, as you might start to sag if too much fat is removed from the area.

Buttocks—Too Small

Ideal Candidate: A woman who's realistic about the outcome. Not everyone can end up with the buttocks of Jennifer Lopez (nor should they!). The best results are usually seen in heavier women with lots of fat to transfer from other parts of the body. But remember, regular weight training and exercise, done properly, are just as likely (if not more so) to give you the desired results.

Procedure: Fat transfer is best option. I am not a fan of buttock implants, as there can be too many complications and they can look terribly fake.

How It's Done: Fat is transferred from one part of body to the buttocks; this procedure is essentially liposuction with the fat then added in another part of the body. This may require two or three procedures.

Pain Factor: Moderate; easily controlled by pain medication.

Recuperation/Downtime: Three to seven days.

How Bad You'll Really Look: Somewhat swollen for one week.

What Could Go Wrong: Infection, poor response to the fat transfer, asymmetry.

When You'll See Results: Immediately.

How Long It Lasts: It should last for a lifetime; however not all the fat always takes (i.e., stays in place without being reabsorbed by the body) after transfer, and repeat transfers may be necessary.

Inside Scoop: Much consideration should be taken before you sign up for this procedure, as you may be very disappointed with the results. Expectations must be realistic because there must be adequate areas of fat elsewhere in the body so that enough can be transferred to the buttocks to make a noticeable difference. If not done correctly, the patient is left with clumps of fat in an irregular pattern, which is not attractive.

Another technique is to use liposuction to reduce the thighs. Many women have an area of fat just below the buttock cheeks of the posterior upper thigh. It's referred to as the "banana roll," as it's shaped like a banana. When that fat is removed, the buttocks automatically look bigger and shapelier.

Calves/Ankles—Too Large or Small

Ideal Candidate: Realistic expectations and good skin quality.

Procedure: Liposuction for large calves/ankles. See Excess Skin—Fat Deposits in Specific Areas.

Inside Scoop: Although implants are an option for those with disproportionately small calves, I don't recommend them. They look fake, the scar is visible, and the implant could dislodge or harden. Better to stick to exercise to bulk up your legs. See Chapter 7.

Excess Skin—Fat Deposits in Specific Areas

Ideal Candidate: Someone at an ideal weight and who exercises regularly but still cannot get rid of well-defined areas of fat.

Procedure: Liposuction, traditional or ultrasonic.

How It's Done: Local anesthetic and saltwater solution is infiltrated in the area, then suctioned out with a canula.

Pain Factor: Moderate, easily controlled with pain medication.

Recuperation/Downtime: Depending on the number of areas treated, five days to two weeks.

How Bad You'll Really Look: Swollen and with modest bruising.

What Could Go Wrong: Over-resection or under-resection in an area causing skin and contour irregularities; pulmonary embolus (blood clot to lung), which is very rare.

When You'll See Results: Four to six weeks after the swelling goes down.

How Long It Lasts: Forever, if there is no weight gain and the patient stays active and exercises. Since fat cells are removed from the area, any extra weight gain after the procedure will not appear in that area.

Inside Scoop: One of the biggest misperceptions I deal with on a nearly daily basis is from patients who think liposuction is a weight-loss tool. They see these stories about people who've had five or six liters of fat sucked out at one time, and they want that for themselves.

Trust me—liposuction is *not* for weight loss! It works best *after* you've lost all your weight. And actually, it works best on those who don't really *need* it, but are dissatisfied with pockets of fat that won't go away despite a healthy weight and active lifestyle. I've had models come to me—young and gorgeous and thin—and they tell me they hate the minuscule pooches on their thighs, and I ask them if they exercise, and of course the answer is no. I tell them that if they went to the gym they'd firm up that area in no time, but then they tell me they have a bathing suit shoot coming up and they'd rather have someone do their work for them. Yep—it's the Super-Downsize Me generation!

It's always a delicate, diplomatic balancing act when a new patient says she wants liposuction when what she really needs to do is lose a small amount of weight or add some muscle tone to her body. Yet I've lost patients when I gently tried to urge them away from surgery when a much less invasive solution is the best option, as there is a lot of natural defensiveness.

Excess Skin—Sagging Skin in Midsection

Ideal Candidate: A person who is close to ideal body weight and exercises regularly; someone who is post-pregnant and not planning on more children; nonsmoker.

Procedure: Tummy tuck.

How It's Done: Excess skin and fat are removed through an incision in the lower abdominal region just above the groin, where the scar can easily be hidden by panties or a bikini. A tightening of abdominal wall with internal sutures corrects laxity in the area.

Pain Factor: Moderate to severe, strong pain medication is a must.

Recuperation/Downtime: Two to six weeks.

How Bad You'll Really Look: Bruised and swollen; drains are usually required for three to seven days.

What Could Go Wrong: Infection, skin loss, bad scar.

When You'll See Results: Immediately, improving as swelling goes down in six to eight weeks.

How Long It Lasts: Lifetime if there is no weight gain or pregnancies.

Inside Scoop: Tummy tucks are a popular "mommy makeover" with a high level of satisfaction afterward. When I do this procedure, I always ask my patients to show me where their bikini line is, so I know where to put the scar so it won't show. Yet one of my tummy tuck patients in her midforties came to see me several months after a flawless procedure, complaining that the scar showed when she wore her low-rider jeans. She was a patient I knew well and could joke with, and I said, "What the heck are you wearing low-riders for—are you raiding your daughter's closet?" She laughed for a long time.

Excess Skin—Weight Loss

Ideal Candidate: Weight loss is complete, and weight has also reached a plateau and has been stable for six months; highly motivated nonsmoker in good health.

Procedure: Abdominoplasty or belt abdominoplasty (where excess skin is removed circumferentially), thigh lift, or body lift.

How It's Done: Excess skin and fat is cut away, leaving a long scar on the lower abdomen, thighs, and/or lower back.

Pain Factor: High; strong pain medication is a must.

Recuperation/Downtime: Two to eight weeks.

How Bad You'll Really Look: Bruised and swollen, plus you'll usually require drains for a week or more.

What Could Go Wrong: Poor scarring, infection, hematoma, or seroma.

When You'll See Results: Immediately, with even more improvement as swelling gradually goes down.

How Long It Lasts: It lasts a lifetime, as long as patients maintain their weight.

Inside Scoop: There is a high level of satisfaction with these operations. These patients have gone to extraordinary measures (surgery or strict diet and exercise) to achieve significant weight loss but are then left with truly deforming layers of redundant skin. Although this surgery will always leave significant scars, the dramatic change in body contour overrides them (many of the scars can be hidden by clothing or even properly selected bathing suits). Often, the surgery must be done in stages, and in the case of massive weight loss, may require as many as three stages and smaller touch-up procedures down the road.

Hands—Crepey/Thin/Mottled Skin

Procedure: Hand lifts are technically feasible, but I've never done one and cannot recommend it.

Inside Scoop: Using lasers or chemicals peels to rejuvenate the hand's tender skin are much better options, as is fat transfer to the back of the hands to increase volume and rejuvenate them, as described in Appendix B. The results are immediate and downtime is only one or two days.

Exercises

The exercises in this chapter have been created by personal trainer Jill Livoti, certified by the Aerobics and Fitness Association of America (AFAA) and International Sports Sciences Association (ISSA), and she takes continuing education classes under the aegis of National Academy of Sports Medicine (NASM) and American Council on Exercise (ACE) as well. She is also a national title-holding bodybuilder and choreographer. Jill designed these exercises to target specific areas, but you should consider them to be part of a larger workout program.

A few tips to make exercising even more productive:

- Always do a warm-up first for about 5–10 minutes. This will help get the blood flowing. If you're at home, you can jump rope, walk up and down stairs, march or run in place, do jumping jacks, or mix it all up. If you're at the gym, use the treadmill, elliptical machines, StairMaster, or bicycles.

- A set is a chosen exercise or exercises done for a number of repetitions for a certain number of times. Start with 2 sets and build up to 3 or 4.

- Reps, or repetitions, are the number of times you perform an exercise. Start with 5–10 and build up to 12–20. When 20 is too easy, increase the weight of the dumbbell.

- If you're a beginner, you might want to pick one exercise per muscle group at first. Start slow. Try 5–10 reps and 1–2 sets.

Exercises for Abdominals and Core

Every woman will benefit from a strong core. Toned abs will automatically improve your posture, relieve stress on your back muscles, and help you look slimmer.

Abdominal work is one area where Jill often sees people in the gym doing the wrong thing. Many do their crunches on a large exercise ball, which can be great—but only if you know what you're doing. You should always start on the floor, and move on to more advanced skills after several weeks of regular exercising.

And you don't need to do crunches every day. The abdominal muscles need rest just like every other muscle group in your body. If you're a beginner, do a pattern of exercises one day, rest two days. Work it up to two days of exercise, followed by one day of rest; then progress to three days of exercise, one day of rest.

These exercises can be done at home or in the gym. Be sure to use a mat.

Crunch

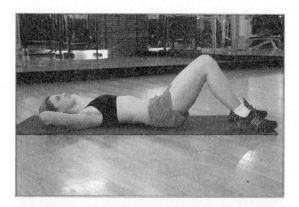

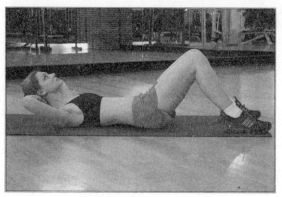

To be done at home or in the gym:

1. Lie on your back, looking up at the ceiling.

2. Bend your knees and keep your feet flat.

3. Lace your fingertips lightly at the back of your head and neck. Do not pull your head with your hands, or you won't be engaging your abs muscles properly.

4. With your eyes looking toward the ceiling, keep a space between your chin and your chest, about the size of an orange.

5. Exhale. Lift your shoulders off the ground and lift them up.

6. Push your belly button into the floor. Hold.

7. Inhale while slowly lowering your shoulders down until they almost touch the mat.

8. Repeat.

Facedown Plank

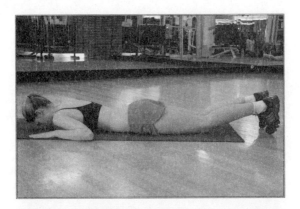

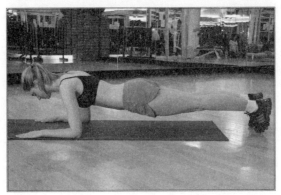

To be done at home or in the gym:

1. Lie face down on a mat.

2. Place your forearms and elbows on the mat with your shoulders and elbows at a 90-degree angle.

3. Push yourself up on your feet to form a plank.

4. Keep your abs tight and back flat. Do not lift your hips or butt. Keep an even line.

5. Try to hold the plank for 10 seconds. When stronger, increase to 20 seconds.

6. Repeat.

Exercises for the Arms

It's especially important to tone both the biceps as well as the triceps.

Biceps—Concentration Curl

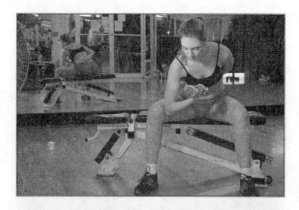

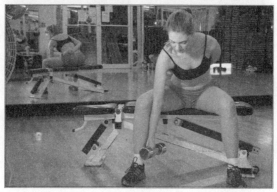

To be done at home or in the gym:

1. Sit on a chair or bench.

2. Bend your upper body forward, keeping your abs tight at all times.

3. Pick up a dumbbell and place your elbows tight to your knees or inner thighs. The arm holding the dumbbell should be fully extended.

4. Exhale as you bring the dumbbell toward your shoulders, about 2–3 inches away. Squeeze the biceps muscle.

5. Inhale as you lower the dumbbell to the start position.

6. Repeat.

7. Switch sides.

8. Repeat.

Biceps—Barbell Curl

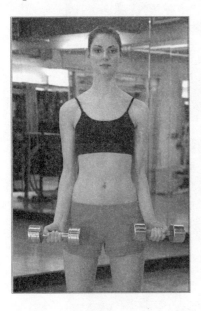 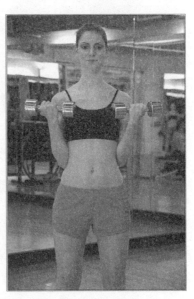

To be done at home or in the gym:

1. Grasp a barbell (if at the gym) or dumbbells (if at home) with an underhand grip.

2. Stand with your feet hip-width apart, abs tight, with a slight bend in your knees.

3. Keep your elbows tight to your sides. Do not bend your wrists.

4. Exhale and bend your elbows, bringing the barbell or dumbbells toward your shoulders.

5. Inhale as you slowly return to the start position.

6. Repeat.

Triceps—Lying Triceps Extension

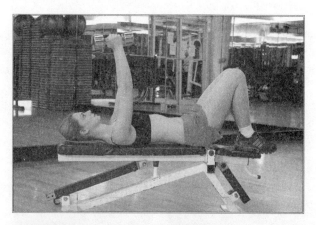

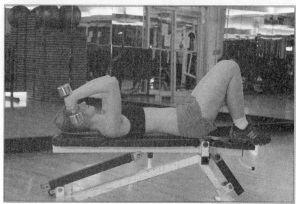

To be done at home or in the gym:

1. Lie on the floor or a bench, looking up at the ceiling with your feet flat on the floor.

2. Grab a dumbbell in each hand and hold straight above your shoulders. Keep your upper arms still.

3. Exhale as you bend at the elbows and lower the dumbbells toward your ears or forehead. Watch your wrists—you do not want to bend them.

237

4. Inhale as you slowly return the dumbbells to the start position, just shy of locking your elbows.

5. Repeat.

Triceps—Triceps Push-down

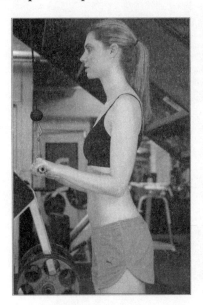 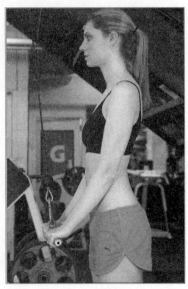

To be done in the gym with a cable pulley:

1. Stand with your feet hip-width apart.

2. Face the high cable pulley.

3. Grab the straight bar, which attaches to the cable. Keep your palms down and elbows tight to your sides.

4. Exhale and press the bar down by straightening your arms, so the bar almost touches your thighs. Don't snap your elbows.

5. Hold for a second, and then inhale and return to an L position with your elbows.

6. Repeat.

Exercises for the Back (and Posture)

As a surgeon, I do have a tendency to hunch over, so Jill insists that I do the kind of back work in the gym (exercises like lat [latissimus back muscle] pull-downs and seated cable rows) to strengthen all the muscles around my spinal column and hips so that I stand properly during surgery. And then she kills me with the abdominal work, since when you train correctly, your abdominal muscles will automatically be engaged.

Since she started working with me many years ago, I've come to appreciate that strong back muscles will automatically allow me to stand up straighter and have a flatter belly, too.

One-Arm Dumbbell Row

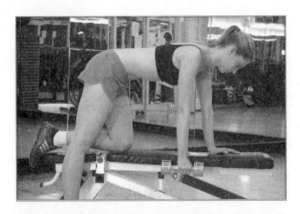

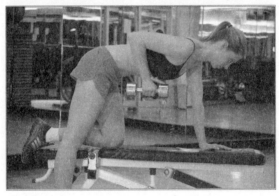

To be done at home with hand weights or on a bench at the gym:

1. Place your left knee and left hand on a bench.

2. Grab the dumbbell with your right hand.

3. Keep your back flat, head straight, and spine aligned.

4. Using your shoulder blades and back muscles, exhale and pull your right elbow up until the dumbbell is almost touching your rib. (It will look like you're sawing wood.)

5. Squeeze, and then inhale as you slowly return the weight to the start position.

6. Repeat.

7. Repeat on other side.

Lat Pull-down

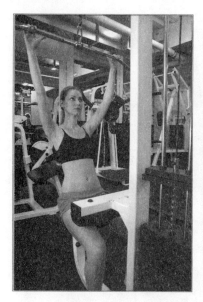
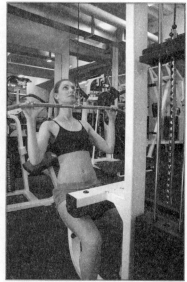

To be done in the gym with a lat machine:

1. Adjust the seat of the machine so you fit snugly under the pads.

2. Grasp the wide bar and sit facing the cable. Place your hands in the bend of the bar. Your arms should be fully extended and comfortable.

3. Lean back a little and engage your abs.

4. Exhale as you pull the bar down to your upper chest (about an inch or two away from your clavicle). Make sure you squeeze your shoulder blades.

5. Inhale as you slowly return to the start position.

6. Repeat.

Seated Cable Row

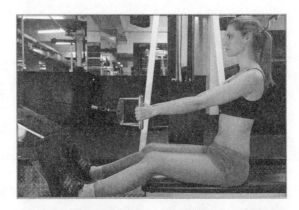

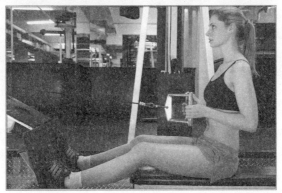

To be done in the gym with a cable row machine:

1. Sit up tall, facing the cable row with your feet on the foot plate.

2. Keep your knees slightly bent (so this exercise will be joint friendly!).

3. Grasp the grip handle. Stay tall and keep your abs tight.

4. Exhale as you pull the handle toward your midsection.

5. Squeeze your shoulder blades. Keep your elbows tight to your body. Do not round your back or bend your wrists.

6. Inhale as you return to start position.

7. Repeat.

Exercises for the Buttocks, Hips, and Thighs

Any exercises that work the large group of gluteus muscles will improve the shape of your derriere. Regular cardiovascular exercise is also a powerful tool for improving your appearance. It may make excess skin less significant, as larger muscles will fill out the region. Fat cells may not disappear, but if you replace slack areas with firm muscle, you will definitely make a difference, especially if you add weight training that further firms your muscles.

If the shape of your buttocks is flat, doing squats will help, but you need to do a different range of repetitions than those that shrink large buttocks. To gain mass, you should use a higher weight level and fewer reps. To lose mass, you should do more reps with less weight.

Two buttocks-improving exercises you cannot do without are lunges and squats. Leg lifts also help a lot. If you're not going to a gym, you'll see faster results if you add light ankle weights or use resistance bands, which are very inexpensive.

Even if you're not in the middle of an exercise routine, you can add walking lunges to your daily routine whenever you move around the house. Or simply walk slowly up and down the stairs, with soup cans in your hands for added weight.

If you have troublesome knees that are bothered by lunges, you can do leg lifts or pelvic tilts on the floor.

Use a padded mat underneath your feet to minimize any joint strain.

Pelvic Tilt

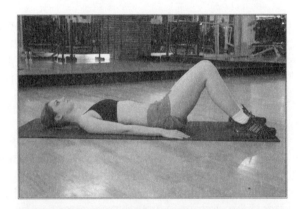

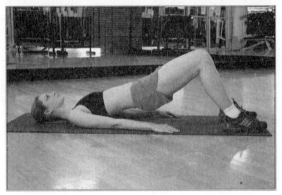

To be done at home or in the gym:

1. Lie on your back.

2. Keep your head straight, looking up at the ceiling, and your back flat.

3. Squeeze your butt and lift your hips toward the ceiling.

4. Keep your back straight. Don't strain. Hold for a second squeeze.

5. Lower slowly.

6. Repeat.

Squat

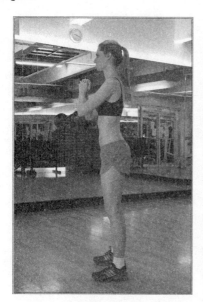 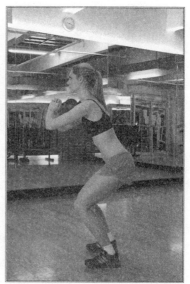

To be done at home or in the gym:

1. Stand with your feet shoulder-width apart. Keep your head forward and your abs tight.

2. Sit back as if you are sitting down into a chair. (You can use a sturdy chair if you like.) Do not let your knees move forward over your toes. Press down through your heels, and keep your hips back. Don't go too far down, and do not arch your back.

3. Squeeze your butt for a moment.

4. Slowly return to an almost standing straight position. Do not lock your knees.

5. Repeat.

Step-up

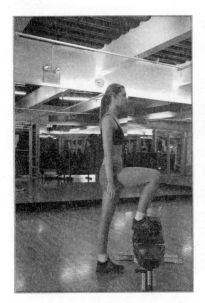 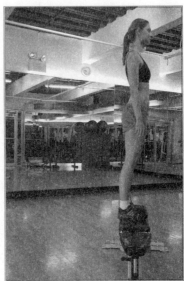

To be done at home or in the gym:

1. Step up on a stair (or bench, stool, step) with your right foot.

2. Using your abs, legs, and butt, squeeze and pull up your left leg and foot to the stair, touch it, and return that left foot to the floor. Mix up the pace. Do some fast reps and then some slow ones.

3. Repeat.

4. Switch legs.

5. Repeat.

Lunge

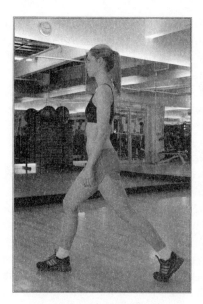 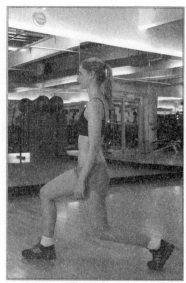

To be done at home or in the gym:

1. Holding a dumbbell in each hand, or with hands on hips, stand with your feet hip-width apart.

2. Take a large step forward with your right leg. Make sure your knee is not going over your toes.

3. Bend both knees until the front thigh is parallel to the ground.

4. Your back knee is should go down about 2–3 inches from the floor. Never let that back knee touch the ground. (Beginners should only go down as far as they feel comfortable.)

5. Slowly return to the start position. Almost lock your knee—but not quite, as you want to keep tension in the muscle.

6. Repeat.

7. Switch sides.

8. Repeat.

Exercises for the Chest Area

These will firm the muscles around your breasts and help your posture, too. You will find that doing cardiovascular work combined with healthier eating should have some effect on your breasts as well, as breast tissue is primarily composed of fat.

Jill is a huge fan of push-ups, as they're one exercise that anyone can do, practically anywhere. A push-up is one of those great exercises where many different muscle groups (the abdominals, shoulders, triceps, and secondary muscles) are worked at once, using only the force of your own body weight for resistance. But many women, instantly reminded of their old gym classes and all the unhappy memories about body image, are reluctant to do them. Jill has had clients literally burst into tears when accomplishing their first set of push-ups, because they were able to break through a barrier that had told them they just couldn't do it.

Do as many push-ups as you can—with good form. If that means one at first, one is better than none. As soon as your arms and shoulders become stronger, you'll increase the amount. Don't give yourself an arbitrary number goal. Listen to your body. When doing push-ups becomes easy, crank up the amount, and do them a little bit slower.

If you're not used to push-ups, start on your knees, and eventually move up to a regular push-up done on your toes.

Push-up

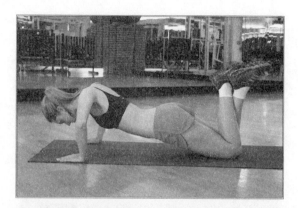

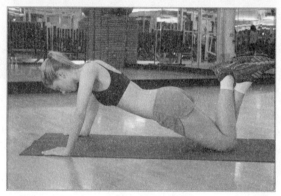

To be done at home or in the gym:

1. Begin on your knees. Place your hands about shoulder width apart (too close and they will work your triceps, not your pectorals).

2. Your body should be straight, like a plank.

3. Pull your abs in tight and secure.

4. Inhale as you lower your body slowly to the floor. Don't go too low, as you don't want to stress your shoulders or elbow joints.

5. Exhale as you push your body up.

6. Repeat.

Incline Dumbbell Press

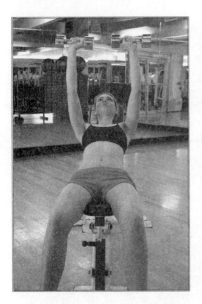 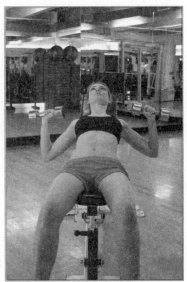

To be done in the gym on an incline bench:

1. The incline press will definitely improve your décolleté and strengthen your shoulders too. So you'll have a better-looking chest area as well as improved posture.

2. Sit on an incline bench at about 45 degrees.

3. Hold a pair of dumbbells with your arms bent almost in your armpits, about an inch away from your shoulders.

4. Exhale and raise the dumbbells toward the center of your chest as you straighten your arms, making a triangle.

5. Squeeze in the center. Don't lock your elbows, and don't hold your breath.

6. Return to the start position in a slow controlled manner.

7. Repeat.

Exercises for the Shoulders

These will strengthen your shoulders, giving you the illusion of a smaller waist and bigger breasts. They'll also improve posture.

Shoulder Press

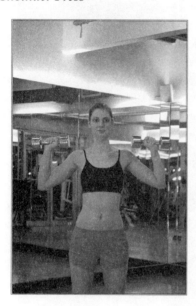 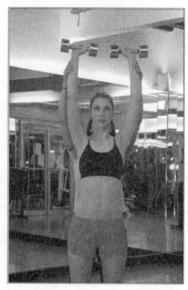

To be done at home or in the gym. If doing at home, you can use soup cans or dumbbells; use a cable or dumbbells in the gym.

1. Stand with a slight bend in your knees, feet shoulder-width apart depending on your comfort level.

2. Make sure your abs are tight and your back is straight, with your head forward.

3. With a dumbbell in each hand, palms forward, place your arms just an inch or two above your shoulders.

4. Exhale and press dumbbells toward the ceiling, bringing your hands close together.

5. Squeeze for a moment and then inhale as you slowly return to start position.

6. Repeat.

Side Lateral Raise

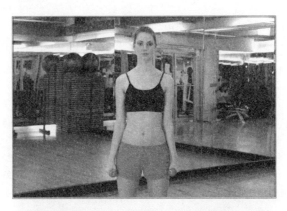

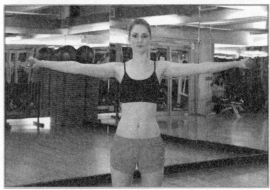

To be done at home or in the gym:

1. Stand with a slight bend in your knees, feet shoulder-width apart depending on your comfort level.

2. Grab a dumbbell in each hand, facing your sides, palms down toward your hips. Keep your head straight and your neck relaxed.

3. Exhale slowly and raise your arms to shoulder level. Keep a slight bend in your elbows to protect your elbow joints.

4. Inhale as you slowly return to start position.

5. Repeat.

Resources

Hair and Makeup

Great Hair: Secrets to Looking Fabulous and Feeling Beautiful Every Day by Nick Arrojo (St. Martin's Griffin, 2008)

Face Forward by Kevyn Aucoin (Little, Brown, 2000)

Making Faces by Kevyn Aucoin (Little, Brown, 1999)

The Art of Makeup by Kevyn Aucoin (Perennial Currents, 1996)

Bobbi Brown: Living Beauty by Bobbi Brown (Springboard Press, 2007)

Fashion in Hair: The First Five Thousand Years by Richard Corson (Peter Owen, 2000)

Makeup: The Art of Beauty by Linda Mason (Watson-Guptill, 2007)

Makeup Your Mind by Francois Nars (powerHouse Books, 2002)

Self-Help/Empowerment

The Six Pillars of Self-Esteem by Nathaniel Branden (Bantam, 1995)

Chicken Soup for the Soul by Jack Canfield, Mark Victor Hansen (HCI, 2001)

How to Enjoy Your Life and Your Job by Dale Carnegie (Pocket Books, 1990)

How to Stop Worrying and Start Living by Dale Carnegie (Pocket Books, rev. ed., 2004)

How to Win Friends and Influence People by Dale Carnegie (Pocket Books, reprint, 1998)

The Quick and Easy Way to Effective Speaking by Dale Carnegie (Pocket Books, 1990)

The Seven Spiritual Laws to Success: A Pocketbook Guide to Fulfilling Your Dreams by Deepak Chopra (Amber-Allen Publishing, 2007)

Buddha: A Story of Enlightenment by Deepak Chopra (HarperOne, 2008)

The 7 Habits of Highly Effective People by Stephen R. Covey (Free Press, 2004)

Eat Pray Love by Elizabeth Gilbert (Penguin Books, 2007)

Emotional Intelligence: 10th Anniversary Edition; Why it Can Matter More Than IQ by Daniel Goleman (Bantam, 2006)

Peace Is Every Step: The Path of Mindfulness in Everyday Life by Thich Nhat Hanh (Bantam, 1992)

The Art of Power by Thich Nhat Hanh (HarperOne, 2008)

How to See Yourself as You Really Are by Dalai Lama (Atria, 2007)

The Blessings of a Skinned Knee: Using Jewish Teachings to Raise Self-Reliant Children by Wendy Mogel (Scribner, reprint, 2008)

How to Be Your Own Best Friend by Mildred Newman and Bernard Berkowi, with Jean Owen (Ballantine, 1986)

Zen and the Art of Motorcycle Maintenance: An Inquiry into Values by Robert M. Pirsig (Harper Perennial Modern Classics, 2008)

Senses and Scent

A Natural History of the Senses by Diane Ackerman (Vintage, 1991)

Aphrodite: A Memoir of the Senses by Isabel Allende (HarperCollins, 1998)

What the Nose Knows: The Science of Scent in Everyday Life by Avery Gilbert (Crown, 2008)

Scent by Annick Le Guerer (Trafalgar Square, 1992)

The Scent of Desire: Discovering our Enigmatic Sense of Smell by Rachel Herz (Harper Perennial, 2008)

The Secret of Scent: Adventures in Perfume and the Science of Smell by Luca Turin (Harper Perennial, 2007)

Style and Fashion

Richard Avedon: Photographs 1946–2004 by Richard Avedon (Louisiana Museum of Modern Art, 2007)

Woman in the Mirror: 1945–2004 by Richard Avedon (Harry N. Abrams, 2005)

Lillian Bassman by Lillian Bassman, Martin Harrison, Catherine Chermayeff, Kathy McCarver Mnuchin, and Nan Richardson (Bullfinch Press, 1997)

The Glass of Fashion by Cecil Beaton (Cassell, 1989)

Halston by Steven Bluttal (Phaidon Press, 2001)

Doing It with Style by Quentin Crisp (Watts, 1981)

The Little Black Book of Style by Nina Garcia (Collins Living, 2007)

Model: The Ugly Business of Beautiful Women by Michael Gross (Harper, 2003)

The Way We Wore: Styles of the 1930s and '40s and Our World Since Then by Marsha Hunt (Fallbrook, 1993)

Annie Leibovitz: Photographs Portfolio 1970–1990 (Stern Portfolio of Photography) by Annie Leibovitz (Te Neues, 1999)

Chanel: A Woman of Her Own by Axel Madsen (Henry Holt, 1991)

New York Fashion by Caroline Rennolds Milbank (Harry N. Abrams, 1996)

Horst Portraits: 60 Years of Style by Terence Pepper, Horst P. Horst, and Charles Saumarez Smith (Harry N. Abrams, 2001)

Scavullo on Beauty by Francesco Scavullo (Vintage Books, 1979)

Mario Testino: Portraits by Mario Testino (Bulfinch, 2002)

D.V. by Diana Vreeland (Da Capo, 2003)

Index

Note: Page numbers in *italics* include photographs/captions.

Acknowledgments

The idea for this book, my first, was hatched over lunch one pretty fall afternoon near Gramercy Park. My friend and attorney, Kerry Smith, invited me to join her and publicist Mary Lengle. Ideas were flying by the time coffee was served. Mary then introduced me to Dana Bacher, my literary agent, and the premise of the book became solidified over another lunch meeting. I owe these three women an enormous debt of gratitude for convincing me that my philosophy and premise regarding the beauty of women, and ultimately the BQ Formula, was a worthy literary endeavor. This book simply would not *be* without these incredibly smart and vivacious ladies.

Karen Moline was a pleasure to work with. Our collaboration was enormously enjoyable and informative for me, and her slant to many aspects of the book was essential to the wonderful flow of the work. She taught me so much about composition and written communication. Her skills are special.

I must thank the staff at Hay House for believing in me and providing their wisdom and support during the project. Reid Tracy furnished inspiration and counsel, and I am most grateful. My editors, Patty Gift and Laura Koch, were incredibly patient with this fledgling author, and their guidance was crucial and so outstanding. Copy editor Melanie Gold made me realize the importance of this facet of the book. The art department at Hay House provided a gorgeous layout for the cover and the rest of the book, complementing the content elegantly. The publicity, sales, and marketing departments have been instrumental in getting out the word about the book.

I would like to thank Dr. Philip Orbuch and Dr. Rena Brand, two of this city's preeminent dermatologists, for their input and assistance regarding content and allowing me to pick their brains with regard to the cutting edge of skin care.

Special thanks to Dr. Ken Bacher, mathematician extraordinaire, for his invaluable help in providing a logical manner to score the BQ quiz.

Jill Livoti, my expert personal trainer, whose dedication to healthy fitness is unyielding. Her contribution to the book was vital and much appreciated.

Thank you Michael Valenti, hair expert, stylist, and dear friend, for assisting Valerie and me with the chapter regarding hair styles and color.

Thanks to Paige Amans and the creative folks at *Looking Your Best* for putting together a sensational Website for the book, www.thebeautyquotientformula.com.

My exceptional office staff, whose patience and allegiance is unparalleled, must be mentioned here. Kimberly Wepner, Cynthia Syamsul, Fabiola Deslouches, Maria Sarmiento, and Pamela Hardial all provided an enormous amount of assistance in various ways to help make this project happen, and I thank you.

To my beautiful Valerie, who reminds me every day that one's BQ truly comes from the heart and her extraordinary radiance grows with each day that we spend together. To my boys, Massimo and Luca, who keep me grounded and remind me daily that I am, indeed, bald!

To my mother Rose, for teaching me to honor and respect women, and to appreciate all of the qualities that come together to make a woman beautiful, inside and out.

Finally, to my father, Dr. Paul Tornambe, who passed away a few years ago, for being the perfect role model to emulate as a physician and more importantly as a person. He taught me to treat my patients as if they were my family and never ever forget that compassion can be as powerful as a prescription.

About the Author

New York City plastic surgeon **Robert M. Tornambe, M.D.,** is a fellow of the American College of Surgeons (F.A.C.S.) and diplomate of the American Board of Plastic Surgery (board certified). In addition to completing his plastic surgery training at the University of Texas–Houston, Dr. Tornambe has completed fellowship training in surgery of the breast with world-renowned plastic surgeons and acted as the chief of the division of plastic surgery at Cabrini Medical Center in New York City for nearly two decades.

Dr. Tornambe has lectured in the United States and Europe and is considered an expert in cosmetic facial and breast surgery. He was listed in *New York Magazine*'s "The Best Doctors in New York." Dr. Tornambe has appeared on *Dateline*, the *Today* show, and *The Charlie Rose Show*; and he was the only New York City–based plastic surgeon to appear on the ABC series *Extreme Makeover*.

Website: **www.thebeautyquotient.com**

Hay House Titles of Related Interest

YOU CAN HEAL YOUR LIFE, the movie,
starring Louise L. Hay & Friends
(available as a 1-DVD program and an expanded 2-DVD set)
Watch the trailer at: **www.LouiseHayMovie.com**

THE SHIFT, the movie,
starring Dr. Wayne W. Dyer
(available as a 1-DVD program and an expanded 2-DVD set)
Watch the trailer at: **www.DyerMovie.com**

▦ ▦ ▦

*COMPLEXION PERFECTION! Your Ultimate Guide to Beautiful Skin
by Hollywood's Leading Skin Health Expert,* by Kate Somerville

*THE CORE BALANCE DIET: 4 Weeks to Boost Your
Metabolism and Lose Weight for Good,* by Marcelle Pick,
MSN, OB/GYN NP, with Genevieve Morgan

FACE IT: What Women Really *Feel As Their Looks Change,*
by Vivian Diller, Ph.D., with Jill Muir-Sukenick

*PERSONAL DEVELOPMENT FOR SMART PEOPLE:
The Conscious Pursuit of Personal Growth,* by Steve Pavlina

*RECIPES FOR HEALTH BLISS: Using NatureFoods & Lifestyle
Choices to Rejuvenate Your Body & Life,* by Susan Smith Jones, Ph.D.

All of the above are available at your local bookstore,
or may be ordered by contacting Hay House (see next page).

▦ ▦ ▦

We hope you enjoyed this Hay House book. If you'd like to receive our online catalog featuring additional information on Hay House books and products, or if you'd like to find out more about the Hay Foundation, please contact:

Hay House, Inc., P.O. Box 5100, Carlsbad, CA 92018–5100

(760) 431-7695 or **(800) 654-5126**
(760) 431-6948 (fax) or **(800) 650-5115 (fax)**
www.hayhouse.com® • **www.hayfoundation.org**

Published and distributed in Australia by: Hay House Australia Pty. Ltd., 18/36 Ralph St., Alexandria NSW 2015 • *Phone:* 612-9669-4299 • *Fax:* 612-9669-4144 www.hayhouse.com.au

Published and distributed in the United Kingdom by: Hay House UK, Ltd., 292B Kensal Rd., London W10 5BE • *Phone:* 44-20-8962-1230 • *Fax:* 44-20-8962-1239 www.hayhouse.co.uk

Published and distributed in the Republic of South Africa by: Hay House SA (Pty), Ltd., P.O. Box 990, Witkoppen 2068 • *Phone/Fax:* 27-11-467-8904 info@hayhouse.co.za • www.hayhouse.co.za

Published in India by: Hay House Publishers India, Muskaan Complex, Plot No. 3, B-2, Vasant Kunj, New Delhi 110 070 • *Phone:* 91-11-4176-1620 *Fax:* 91-11-4176-1630 • www.hayhouse.co.in

Distributed in Canada by: Raincoast, 9050 Shaughnessy St., Vancouver, B.C. V6P 6E5 • *Phone:* (604) 323-7100 • *Fax:* (604) 323-2600 • www.raincoast.com

Take Your Soul on a Vacation

Visit **www.HealYourLife.com®** to regroup, recharge, and reconnect with your own magnificence. Featuring blogs, mind-body-spirit news, and life-changing wisdom from Louise Hay and friends.

Visit **www.HealYourLife.com** today!

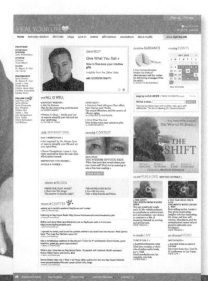

For a complete selection of Hay House products, visit: **www.hayhouse.com**®

Yes, I'd like to receive:

☐ Information on the Wisdom Community

☐ Information on Dr. Christiane Northrup's Women's Wisdom Circle

☐ A Hay House Catalog

Name _____

Address _____

City _____ State _____ Zip _____

Phone _____

PLUS, if you give us your e-mail address, we will e-mail you a $10 coupon good for your online purchase at: **www.hayhouse.com**!

E-mail _____

Take Your Soul on a Vacation!

Visit **www.HealYourLife.com**®, featuring healing news, and life-changing wisdom from your favorite Hay House authors.

Tune in to Hay House Radio to listen to your favorite authors:

HayHouseRadio.com®

To:

HAY HOUSE, INC.
P.O. Box 5100
Carlsbad, CA 92018-5100

Place
Stamp
Here